THE GREAT CATTLE PLAGUE

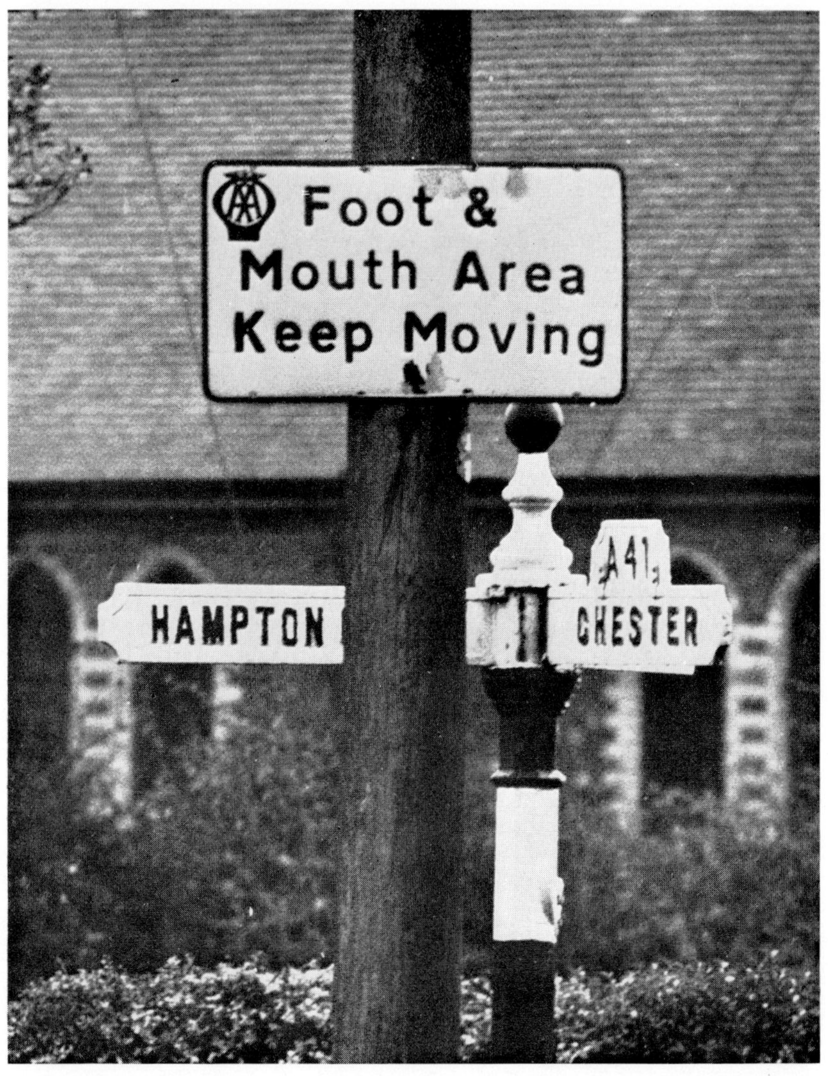

A sign at Whittington, near Oswestry, that became all too familiar during the epidemic.
The Field

THE GREAT CATTLE PLAGUE

An Account of the Foot-and-Mouth Epidemic of 1967-8

by Ralph Whitlock
Farming Correspondent of 'The Field'

with plates and diagrams

JOHN BAKER
5 Royal Opera Arcade, Pall Mall
London SW1

First published in 1968 by
John Baker Publishers Ltd
5 Royal Opera Arcade, Pall Mall
London SW1

SBN 212 99822 6

Printed in Great Britain by
Morrison & Gibb Ltd
London and Edinburgh

Contents

PLATES

TABLES

[1]

Precedents

It is tempting to suppose that foot-and-mouth disease must have been included in the "murrains" which played havoc with British livestock throughout the Middle Ages. Winter mortality rates among cattle and sheep apparently ran as high as 70 per cent in bad years. A sixteenth-century writer, Fitzherbert, describes how an infected manor would stick the head of a dead cow or sheep on a pole in a hedge by the nearest highway, as a warning to drovers and others, which indicates that "murrain" was even then regarded as infectious.

To attempt to identify "murrain" as foot-and-mouth disease, pleuro-pneumonia or any other specific disease is, however, futile. The term included any fatal disease of livestock. Stow, also in the sixteenth century, remarks that even piglets that were eaten by their mothers were reckoned to have succumbed to "murrain".

Foot-and-mouth disease was first officially recorded, or recognised and described identifiably, in August, 1839. The outbreak occurred in one of those large dairy herds which, in the pre-railway age, supplied London with milk. The herd's veterinary surgeon, a Mr Hill, of Islington, sent a detailed report on the symptoms to the Royal Veterinary College.

The attention it attracted and the devastation it caused support the view that this was indeed the first case of the disease to occur in Britain. At the time it was widely supposed to

9

have been introduced from the Continent, and that view is probably correct. It certainly caught the London dairymen unawares. Over 500 animals are said to have been infected in the herd in which it was first noted. Within a month it was present in London's Smithfield market, and before the end of the year it had spread all over the country, including Scotland.

Apparently an epidemic raged throughout most of 1840 and 1841 but then petered out in 1842. Thereafter its incidence was intermittent.

A flare-up occurred in 1845 and 1846, and a much larger one in 1852. Then followed a period of quiescence until 1861, when another epidemic raged. This did not die down until 1865, after which very few cases were reported till 1869, when a new epidemic started. From this time onwards statistics are available. In 1870, 27,354 cases occurred; in 1871, the score was 53,164. Clearly something drastic would have to be done about it.

The reason why we have more detailed information after 1869 is that in that year a Contagious Diseases (Animals) Act was passed, which made outbreaks of foot-and-mouth disease notifiable. So records were kept. It also foreshadowed the control arrangements which still prevail, but with the important difference that it was left entirely to the local authorities to enforce them. The local authorities had power to appoint inspectors, they could prohibit the movement of animals, and they could order someone to go around infected buildings with the disinfectant brush.

They could, but they didn't. In the ensuing years there was a stream of complaints that the rules were not being observed. The trouble was that the Act said what the authorities could do, not what they must do. By 1873 Parliament had decided that the scheme was unworkable so that it might as well be dropped.

Such a defeatist attitude prompted strong protests, notably one from the Royal Agricultural Society of England, so again the House of Commons changed its mind. The new Act which resulted, the Contagious Diseases (Animals) Act of 1878, made the same mistake as its predecessor. It was permissive rather than compulsory. The local authorities were given wider powers, but they were not obliged to use them.

The pattern of future legislation was, however, present. The local authorities could slaughter infected animals and pay compensation for them. But they were not entirely their own masters. They had, if they wished to take such irrevocable action, to report to the Privy Council, who could make an Order accordingly.

Such Orders, under the 1878 Act, were in due course obtained. In 1884 a Slaughter Order was extended to include animals that had been in contact with the disease, as well as those actually infected. The Privy Council, however, still had to authorise the action, and the owner had the right to appeal. Much damage could obviously be done while the law clanked through its pedestrian procedure. In 1885 the local authorities were given power to act on their own initiative.

As might have been expected, the Orders were not very effective. The scheme suffered from the handicap that each local authority had to find the compensation money for any animals it slaughtered. "And why should we spend £500 on compensation when just over the county boundary, in Westhamptsonshire, they refuse to spend anything?" we can imagine the local councils arguing. Infection takes no account of man-made boundaries.

However, the nineteenth century had by this time provided

some precedents for the campaign against foot-and-mouth disease. After the introduction of foot-and-mouth disease in 1839 two other cattle plagues, one of them of even greater menace, had struck British herds. These were rinderpest, which was apparently brought in with a consignment of cattle from the Baltic in May, 1865, and pleuro-pneumonia, which seems to have come from Holland via Ireland about 1840.

Rinderpest struck like a tornado. Between its introduction in May, 1865, and its final disappearance in September, 1867, it is said to have claimed well over 400,000 victims. This is almost certainly short of the mark. The figure was given to the Royal Agricultural Society of England by Lord Cathcart, who admitted that in the densely-populated dairying county of Cheshire the mortality rate was well over 50 per cent as against about 7 per cent for the county as a whole.

After a lot of political shilly-shallying, a Cattle Diseases Prevention Bill was pushed through Parliament on February 20th, 1866. It compelled the slaughter of all infected animals, gave discretionary powers about the slaughter of animals that had been in contact with the disease, and imposed restrictions on the movements of animals. It is true that the local authorities were responsible for administering the Act and had to find the compensation money out of the rates. Nevertheless, there was this compulsory slaughter, and it worked. It took just over eighteen months to clear rinderpest out of the country for good.

So effective had been the policy that it was applied immediately when the disease made brief reappearances in the ports of London and Hull on two occasions in the 1870s. Both were effectively stamped on within a very short time. Since then the country has been entirely free from rinderpest.

As for pleuro-pneumonia, Professor Gamgee, one of the

leading lights in the veterinary world at that time and a champion of the policy which beat rinderpest, estimated that in the six years from 1854 to 1860 many more than a million cattle died from the disease. The Contagious Diseases (Animals) Act of 1867 was therefore aimed at pleuro-pneumonia equally with foot-and-mouth disease. And it was naturally based on the experience gained in the rinderpest campaign.

To begin with, action against pleuro-pneumonia suffered from the same impediment as the campaign against foot-and-mouth disease. It was left to the local authorities, who were torn by the conflicting desires to eradicate the diseases and to keep down the rates. In 1890, therefore, Parliament acted in the matter of pleuro-pneumonia. It took away the executive powers from the local authorities and made the Board of Agriculture responsible. Equally important, it voted a sum of £140,000 annually for a fund to provide compensation for slaughtered animals and generally for the eradication of the disease.

Quick success followed. Travelling inspectors were appointed to track down the disease in cowsheds, markets, fairs and slaughterhouses, without regard to county boundaries. When they found a case, they followed it up and, if necessary, insisted on the slaughter of contact animals as well. By 1896 the number of cases was down to seven, and in 1898 it could fairly be claimed that pleuro-pneumonia had been eradicted.

So, within the space of just over twenty years, campaigns against two of the three disastrous cattle plagues that had ravaged the country had been completely successful. It must have seemed to the authorities that they had only to apply the same methods to conquer foot-and-mouth disease.

This they attempted to do. In 1892 the powers of slaughter and the general conduct of the campaign were transferred from the local authorities to the Board of Agriculture, with access to the central fund for compensation, exactly as with pleuro-pneumonia. The passing of this Act coincided with the first outbreak of foot-and-mouth disease for five years. In all 2,083 animals were slaughtered in this epidemic, of which only 530 were cattle (for the provisions of the Orders had now been extended to all cloven-hoofed animals).

Thereafter, the disease lay more or less quiescent till 1911, though with a brief resurgence in 1900 and 1901. By 1912 a new epidemic was raging, affecting sixteen counties and resulting in the slaughter of 10,385 animals. Then it died down again, though there were desultory outbreaks during most of the war years.

In the 1920s it was back in force. Look at the tally of animals slaughtered in the following decade:

1919—	3,463	1925—	20,000
1920—	11,665	1926—	21,000
1921—	2,942	1927—	10,000
1922—	56,000	1928—	11,000
1923—	128,000	1929—	3,000
1924—	89,000	1930—	300

In previous epidemics imported live animals had usually been blamed for bringing the disease into the country, as with rinderpest and pleuro-pneumonia. Now other sources were suspect. An outbreak in 1908 was traced to hay imported from Holland. In 1922–4, suspicion fell on imported hay and straw that had been used for packing horticultural and other produce. When foot-and-mouth disease was discovered on board a ship carrying live animals from Uruguay to London in 1923, the animals were slaughtered and thrown overboard. Infected pig carcases imported from Holland were found to be responsible for an outbreak in Lanarkshire in 1926. Orders were made controlling such hazards, but still the disease contrived to get in.

In our next chapter we shall be discussing the nature of the disease and how it is spread. To complete our story to date, it is sufficient to say that the battle continues without abatement. The successes recorded against rinderpest and pleuropneumonia have not been repeated.

Indeed, from the statistics it could be argued that foot-and-mouth disease has been winning. From 1931 to 1961 the number of animals slaughtered annually was never less than 1,000. In 19 of those 30 years, the number of victims was over 10,000, and the peaks reached were 31,000 in 1937, 59,000 in 1942, 75,000 in 1952, and 70,000 in 1960.

A welcome respite occurred in 1963 and 1964, which were completely free from the disease, and only one outbreak marred the year 1965. 1966 saw 34 outbreaks resulting in 45,251 slaughterings, and then the autumn of 1967 saw the onslaught of the most devastating of all foot-and-mouth epidemics, which is the subject of this book.

[2]

What is Foot-and-Mouth and How is it Spread?

I found it difficult, in the great cattle plague, to satisfy my non-farming friends with technical information about it.

"But what is it?" they persisted. "We know the papers call it foot-and-mouth disease, but what is its proper name? It must be an 'itis' of some sort."

They found it hard to believe that even scientists use, invariably as they do, the apparently non-technical term, "foot-and-mouth disease".

The disease is caused by a virus, of which there are numerous strains. These strains are grouped into three main types, labelled "O", "A" and "C", and three other types, discovered comparatively recently in southern Africa, known as "S.A.T.1" "S.A.T.2" and "S.A.T.3". Even more recent is the discovery of a seventh type, "ASIA 1". Just to make matters more complex, there is a midway grouping between types and strains known as variants. At the time of the Gowers Report (1954) three variants of type "O" had been described, eleven of type "A", and three of type "C". In print they are usually referred to as "O_1", "O_2", "A_4" and so on.

Most of the British outbreaks have been due to the variant "O_1", though some of the exceptionally virulent "A" types have occasionally threatened from eastern Europe. In January,

16

1960, the authorities had a scare when an outbreak only about a mile from the Animal Virus Research Station at Pirbright, in Surrey, proved to be of the type "S.A.T.2". Clearly the infection had come from the Institute, where the virus had been used in experiments, and precautions had to be drastically tightened.

The type responsible for the great epidemic of 1967 was "O_1".

The symptoms are the same, whichever type, variant or strain of the virus is present.

Most prominent are the numerous blisters which form around the feet and mouth. They are obviously very painful to the animal, which produces excessive quantities of foamy saliva, and are accompanied by high fever. The victim cannot eat, for the blisters (or vesicles) are inside the mouth and on the tongue as well as around the lips, and is often so lame that it cannot walk. Indeed, its feet are frequently so painful that it will remain lying down, and pigs will keep up a squealing in anguished protest. Pregnant animals, particularly cows, are very liable to abort, and the milk supply dries up.

The incubation period is anything from one to about thirty days, but usually from three to eight days. The fever is at its height for two or three days. Then the blisters break, the temperature of the sufferer falls to normal, and recovery is fairly rapid. A few animals may die during the fever period, especially if they were in poor health or condition before the onset of the disease, but most will get better. The chief hazard is infection of the sores which are left when the blisters break. If these become septic, there can be severe secondary symptoms, and recovery can be long delayed.

If foot-and-mouth disease were not so extremely contagious, its treatment would not present any great difficulties. In a later chapter we present the evidence of people who have successfully nursed stricken flocks and herds through to renewed health. The disease is, however, the most infectious animal disease known, and, once it gets a foothold, it goes raging away like a forest fire. It is so infectious that the measures which, we have seen, were effective against rinderpest and pleuro-pneumonia have so far failed against it, and yet, paradoxically, they remain the methods which seem to offer the best hope of eventual success. Only the most ruthless tactics can be considered when dealing with this virulent foe.

All cloven-hoofed animals are susceptible to foot-and-mouth. For practical purposes, in Britain these consist of cattle, sheep, pigs and goats, but deer can become infected and act as carriers. So, curiously enough, can hedgehogs and, occasionally, rats. A few instances of human beings suffering from the disease have been known.

In laboratory experiments guinea-pigs, rabbits and mice can be infected, but these animals are not apparently susceptible to natural infection.

Although the virus can only multiply and become effective in the living tissue of a host animal, it can lie dormant for a very long time. Under laboratory conditions, it has been kept alive for many years. It thrives on cold and darkness and can survive on meat kept in cold store for four or five months. Heat and sunlight, on the other hand, quickly destroy it.

Hundreds of millions of viruses exist in the bodies of infected animals and are spread by the animals' urine, dung, milk or saliva or by direct contact. Everything in the vicinity of the victim is therefore liable to become infected, and the fact that the infection can survive for so long on practically every material from buckets to rubber boots make it exceptionally difficult to control.

Once an outbreak occurs, almost any agent may carry it to the neighbours. Birds have long been suspect, and anyone who has watched flocks of starlings moving from an infected farm to an adjacent uninfected one is bound to be influenced by the circumstantial evidence. On the other hand farms in infected areas, over which starlings and other birds have ranged at will, have often remained free.

Circumstantial evidence, too, is strongly in favour of the disease being wind-borne. In the 1967–8 epidemic most of the early outbreaks were in a wedge-shaped territory with the apex at Llanyblodwell, where the first outbreak occurred. After a fortnight or so, the wind, which had been in the south-west, suddenly switched to the north, and within a few days an outbreak had been reported at Spetchley, in Worcestershire, far to the south of the others.

Human boots and clothing, the tyres of vehicles and domestic animals are obvious potential carriers. Our examination of the details of the 1967–8 epidemic, will reveal all manner of other agents. One old farmer swore that the disease was spread by disinfectant! If one reads "disinfectors" for "disinfectant" there is just a chance that he was right.

Of even greater importance than the means by which foot-and-mouth disease is spread from a known infected centre is source of a primary outbreak. We can think of a score of ways by which the infection travelled from Llanyblodwell to the farms of Shropshire and Cheshire, but how on earth did it get to Llanyblodwell in the first place?

In the Report of the Departmental Committee on Foot-and-Mouth Disease, 1952–4, more generally known as the Gowers Report (from its chairman, Sir Ernest Gowers), 540 primary outbreaks occurring between the years 1938 to 1952 were investigated.

Of these, birds were the likely agents of introduction in 88 cases; swill in 214 primary outbreaks; contact with imported meat and bones, other than in swill, in 50; and infected serum in one case. Thirty-six were of unknown origin but possibly through contact with swill; in the remaining 151 outbreaks, the origin was completely obscure. Infected imported meat from South America is, as we shall see, blamed, though again on circumstantia evidence, for the great epidemic of 1967–8.

[3]

Prevention and Control

Measures for prevention and control are necessarily two-pronged.

They are first directed towards preventing primary outbreaks; secondly, towards stopping the spread from and minimising the effects of a primary outbreak.

From the very beginning—that is, from the very first outbreak in 1839—it was realised that foot-and-mouth disease came to this country from overseas. Very sensibly, the importation of susceptible live animals was promptly prohibited. Three years later this legislation was rescinded, and for much of the nineteenth century livestock were imported from the Continent without let or hindrance.

Under the Contagious Diseases (Animals) Act of 1892, which we have already met with, imports of cattle were prohibited from countries in which the disease was present. In that same year an outbreak of foot-and-mouth disease in Islington was traced to cattle brought in from Denmark, which country was promptly put on the banned list. By the end of the year the schedule had twenty-five countries on it. The Diseases of Animals Act of 1896 went even further. It prohibited the import of any animal from a foreign country, save for immediate slaughter, unless specially authorised by the Government. These regulations still prevail. The Government's permission has had to be sought for the importation of Charolais cattle, Landrace pigs and other live-stock by means of which we have sought to improve our flocks and herds since the Second World War.

As fresh sources of infection were established, new regulations were made. For instance, a Glasgow outbreak in February, 1908, was traced to hay brought over from Holland. The result was the issuing of the Foreign Hay and Straw Order of 1908, which prohibited such imports unless the authorities were satisfied that the traffic was perfectly safe. The prohibition has been brought up to date but still operates.

When in the outbreaks of 1922 to 1924 infection was traced to packing material the Foot-and-Mouth Disease (Packing Materials) Order of 1925 was passed. It was reinforced by the Importation of Meat (Wrapping Materials) Order of 1932. The discovery of foot-and-mouth disease infection in imported pig *carcases* from Holland and Belgium in Scotland in 1926 was followed by the introduction of legislation to prohibit the importation of carcases from countries known to be suffering from the disease.

In 1927 a Research Committe made some startling revelations of the length of time the virus could survive in frozen meat—as much as 76 days in bone marrow. An order was quickly drafted to make compulsory the boiling of swill before feeding to animals.

The Ministry of Agriculture deserves high marks for vigilance. As soon as it has spotted a bolt-hole, it has effectively stopped it. At least it has taken the necessary powers to stop it, whenever it wants to. Deplorably, it does not always use those powers.

Let us look again at the Gowers Committee's analysis of the 540 primary outbreaks from 1938 to 1952. Setting aside the one outbreak due to infected serum, the others fall into three groups. In 151 cases the causes were completely obscure; in 88 birds were considered to be the most likely carriers; the remaining 300 were thought to be connected in some way with swill or imported meat or bones.

Among birds, the two favourite scapegoats are starlings and gulls, though almost any migrating bird comes under suspicion. It is estimated that about 120 million birds move into or across Britain on migratory movements twice a year. The tide flows north in spring and south (or rather, south-west) in autumn, though with many eddies and cross-currents. Huge flocks of birds can and do cross the English Channel or the North Sea in a few hours within a single night.

Starlings, in particular, are numerous and gregarious birds which frequent farms. They can be flying around the farm-yard or perched on cows' backs on a farm in Holland or North Germany one day and doing the same on an English farm the next. It has been shown experimentally that the virus of foot-and-mouth disease can remain alive on the feet and feathers of a starling for 91 hours. The virus has also been recovered from the droppings of a starling which ate contaminated material 26 hours earlier. There is no evidence, or even suggestion, that the virus can multiply on birds, but beyond any reasonable doubt a starling could carry the infection across the sea to British farms.

Gulls, too, are regarded with suspicion, especially as, in the present century, they have taken to coming inland regularly to feed on farmland. A Channel or North Sea crossing means nothing to a gull. Gulls are also greedy and omnivorous feeders. They pick up all manner of garbage, including ships' swill, and later regurgitate it. The infection could easily be spread by this means.

The evidence regarding the spread of the 1951–2 epidemic

points strongly to birds as the main agent. The primary outbreaks occurred first in Lincolnshire and then around our eastern and southern coasts to Dorset, keeping time with the spread of the epidemic south-westwards along the opposite shores of the Continent. Most of the primary outbreaks were relatively near the coast.

What then? Starlings and gulls are exceedingly numerous birds. To exterminate them throughout the world, or even in Europe, would be an impossible project. Imagination boggles at the prospects of the international campaign that would be necessary. And even if such a fantastic idea could be made practicable we would have eliminated only a couple of the suspects. Other birds would doubtless increase in numbers to fill the vacuum.

We have been discussing only primary outbreaks. Once foot-and-mouth disease is in the distirct, we can have every sympathy with the farmer who tries to keep flocks of starlings off his land. With this in mind, the Ministry's advice in the 1967–8 epidemic to keep cattle indoors was a sensible precaution. But it was not effective. The herds which were housed in buildings in which every conceivable precaution against infection was taken seemed just as likely to catch the disease as those which remained in the open.

The 88 instances in which the Gowers Committee considered birds to be the probable causes of primary outbreaks comprised 16 per cent of the total in the period under review. We will now look at the 151 cases (or 28 per cent) the origin of which was obscure. Birds may have been involved, of course, and so may have swill or infected meat, but there was no evidence, one way or the other. So it will be useful here to consider the other possible ways by which infection can be spread. There are three main ones:

1. Wind or water
2. Human beings and vehicles
3. Agricultural imports

While wind and water undoubtedly assist in spreading the disease once it becomes established in this country, it is doubtful whether they could be responsible for a primary outbreak. Scandinavian scientists are convinced that a southerly or south-westerly wind can carry the infection from Germany across the sea to the Danish islands and from Denmark to southern Sweden, the virus presumably surviving on minute flecks of saliva or in water droplets. For it to cross the North Sea or the English Channel to Britain, however, seems a very doubtful feat, except perhaps in the neighbourhood of the Straits of Dover, with the wind in exactly the right direction.

Human agency is a much more likely source of primary infection. If the birds are to be condemned because they can travel direct from Continental to British farms, we must also regard with suspicion human beings who make the same journey, and, of course, the vehicles they travel in. Myxomatosis, the rabbit plague, is reliably reported to have travelled to Kent from France on the tyres of cars in 1953, and the equally infectious foot-and-mouth virus could use the same transport. The extraordinary precautions taken by the Irish Government (as described in a later chapter) to prevent travellers bringing the virus across the Irish Sea (they even marooned many of their citizens in England for Christmas) showed how well they recognised the danger. Our own preventive measures have seldom if ever been as drastic or thorough.

The agricultural imports referred to in our third category are chiefly vegetables and seeds, for animal and animal products are treated separately. Theoretically it is possible for the infection to come in in sacks of potatoes or grass seed or in crates of cauliflower, as we have already seen it once did in bales of hay and in straw used for packing. No outbreak has been traced to such sources, however, for a very long time, and the risk is generally felt to be negligible.

We come now to the 300 primary outbreaks (56 per cent) thought to be connected with imported meat and swill. In practice, imported meat and swill amount to the same thing, as we shall realise if we ask ourselves, How does the virus get into the swill? The answer must be: from imported meat.

The problem has been tackled at two levels. The first is the regulation of imports; the second, the treatment of the swill.

To deal with the second of these first, an Order was made in 1927 (and amended in 1957) requiring that all swill shall be boiled for at least one hour. All plants processing kitchen waste now have to be licensed, too, a fact which has tended to cut down the wholesale dodging of the regulations which formerly went on.

The big gap in our defences is now the period between the time when the infected meat, bones or offal are discarded for human consumption and the time when they reach the swill cooker. I don't mean that these items are deliberately discarded because they are known to be infective. No, they are scraps of waste meat, bones thrown out for the dogs, and similar odds and ends. Sometimes they find their way to rubbish dumps, where vermin gnaw at them and spread the disease. The 1967 epidemic is thought to have started from some such source as this.

Whatever the method by which the infection reaches our shores and establishes itself when it gets here, the basic fact is that it must come from overseas. The virus is not a permanent resident in our country. In many European countries it is endemic, but in recent years at a low level. The situation in South America is more serious.

South America is much too far away for birds or the wind to carry the infection to us, but its countries do export large quantities of meat to Britain, and these can constitute a danger which everyone has recognised for a long time. As far back as 1928 an agreement was reached with Argentina and other South American countries over the control measures for meat exports to us.

In theory, these measures are completely adequate. The animals themselves are supposed to have three inspections, one at the farm of origin, one at the market, and one at the abattoir and freezing-plant. Not only the individual animals but the entire farm has to be declared free from the disease. At the abattoir, if one animal of a consignment is found to be infected the whole lot are condemned. All abattoirs, freezing-plants and other places where the animals are collected must, if ever they are found to be infected, be thoroughly cleansed and disinfected before they are used again. Vehicles have to be cleaned and disinfected after every use. When packing the meat, only new packing materials may be used. If all these rules were fully observed, there would be next to no danger of infected meat ever reaching Britain.

But consider the difficulties of putting them into practice. Argentina is a huge country. Foot-and-mouth disease is endemic there, and veterinary inspectors are thin on the ground. An outlying estancia has a hundred beasts to send to market. The veterinary inspector, who has not been able to get around to his place lately, accepts his declaration that it is free from foot-and-mouth disease. In fact, a couple of the animals have caught the disease, unknown to their owner. It is still in the incubation stage and so not apparent. The incubation stage can, as we have seen, last for up to thirty days. In that time the cattle have travelled to Buenos Aires, have been through the abattoir and freezing-plant and are packed up for export to Britain. Inspectors have taken samples all along the route, but they have happened not to hit on these three carcases. And so yet another batch of trouble arrives at our ports.

We must admit that it is not often that contaminated meat slips through the mesh in this way. Otherwise we would be dealing with an endless succession of new outbreaks. On the other hand, our experiences of 1967–8 have taught us how much damage just one infected bone can start.

It is too late. The enemy has crept in. A primary outbreak has occurred. What do we do now?

Farmers in this country are remarkably co-operative. There was a case, earlier in 1967, of a Warwickshire farmer who failed to report an outbreak of foot-and-mouth disease, and for his neglect was fined £400 and described by the judge as "a menace to the community". Almost invariably, however, a farmer who suspects foot-and-mouth disease among his animals immediately informs his veterinary surgeon or the police, regardless of the distress it causes him.

The farmer phones the vet, who, in the case of a primary outbreak, takes a swab and sends it post-haste to the Animal Research Station at Pirbright. While the verdict from the experts is awaited, the vet notifies the police and the Ministry of Agriculture's local office, who straightaway declare the district within a ten-mile radius an infected area. Within this unhallowed circle movement of animals is permitted, on licence, only when urgently necessary—as, for instance, when the cows are grazing in a meadow and have to be moved along a road to their milking parlour. No animals are allowed to move out of the area, on any pretext. Except for fatstock for immediate slaughter, all markets are closed, and even for this purpose markets are prohibited within five miles of an outbreak.

On the infected farm itself, once the disease is confirmed, a state of siege is imposed. No one, except with the written authority of the person in charge, is allowed to enter or leave the premises. Anyone with an unavoidable reason for coming in has to don overalls and rubber boots which are thoroughly disinfected.

Such persons, of course, include those involved in the slaughter of the animals on the farm. Among them are the Ministry's valuers, the veterinary surgeons and the slaughter-men. For their benefit footbaths filled with disinfectant are placed at the entrances to the farm. After the slaughter is completed and the carcases have been disposed of, either by burning or burial, the entire premises are disinfected. The vets and the slaughter team wash their boots, gloves and coats with disinfectant and then depart. A policeman is placed on guard duty at the farm gate, charged with seeing that no one leaves or enters for four days. The farmer and his family are left, isolated, with their thoughts.

If no further outbreak occurs in the district, after fourteen days the size of the infected area is reduced to a radius of five miles. After another week it shrinks to the infected farm and its immediate neighbours. A further seven days sees the end of the emergency.

It is, of course, seldom that a primary outbreak is not followed by other outbreaks in the same district, and a farm can remain in an infected area for months. Complications arise when, as in the 1967 epidemic, a market is involved. The Ministry officials then have the colossal task of tracing every animal that has passed through the market. When an epidemic develops, the Ministry sets up a local centre of operations which is manned day and night. On wall maps the location of every animal in the vicinity of infected premises is marked. A careful watch is kept on flocks and herds likely to be exposed to infection.

Beyond the infected area, or areas, the Ministry can establish a controlled area of any size, in which it can shut markets, control or prohibit the movement of animals and impose any other restrictions that seem advisable. On November 18th, 1967, the whole of England and Wales was declared a controlled area.

[4]

Journal of the Plague Months

The First Attacks

When the first outbreak was confirmed on the farm of Mr
Richard Ellis in the village of Llanyblodwell, Shropshire, on
October 25th, 1967, no one could have guessed at the devastation which was to follow. Comparative immunity from the
disease for a number of years had fostered a sense of security.

The one complicating factor in the Shropshire outbreak was
that it coincided with market day at Oswestry, only a few miles
away. Some 7,000 head of stock were sold there that day,
among them two cows from Mr Ellis's farm.

The Ministry of Agriculture acted quickly. From midnight
on October 25th it declared an area of about ten miles around
Llanyblowell to be an Infected Area, while the usual restriction
of movement of animals was imposed for the counties of
Cheshire, Shropshire, Staffordshire, Montgomeryshire, Denbighshire and Flintshire. Ministry officials then set about the
exacting task of tracing all animals that had passed through
Oswestry market on the crucial day.

By October 30th the task had been completed, and the
Ministry circulated an order removing the standstill restrictions
for the whole area. No harm had been done, it seemed.

Mr Ellis's two cows could not have been carrying the infection. Even as the circular was being posted, however, reports of two further outbreaks came in. One was at Darnhall, near Winsford, in Cheshire—a good thirty-five miles north-east of Llanyblodwell; the other at Borwick, near Carnforth, on the borders of Lancashire and Westmoreland, this being about 110 miles from the original outbreak. No apparent connection existed between any of these three outbreaks.

A new restriction of movement order was placed on the counties of Lancashire, Westmoreland, Cheshire, Cumberland and the West Riding of Yorkshire, while the infected areas around the Shropshire and Cheshire outbreaks were extended to form one large area which included the towns of Shrewsbury, Market Drayton, Crewe, Northwich, Birkenhead, Corwen, Bala and Welshpool.

Such was the position at midnight on October 30th, but thereafter news of fresh outbreaks came thick and fast. Three days later, on November 2nd, the Ministry had confirmed 40 outbreaks, extending over the counties of Shropshire, Cheshire, Denbighshire, Flintshire, Lancashire and Montgomeryshire. By the Saturday evening, November 4th, 4,858 cattle, 4,404 sheep and 1,697 pigs had been slaughtered. Movement of animals had been banned in the whole of northern England and Wales, from Merioneth to the Humber. Over 100 Ministry veterinary surgeons were devoting their time to the epidemic, and a permanent headquarters had been set up in the police station at Oswestry. The stunned and alarmed farmers of the north-west were still wondering what had hit them.

The Ministry of Agriculture had proved almost too efficient. The standstill order on Oswestry market on October 25th was imposed within ten minutes of the confirmation of the disease at Llanyblodwell. In consequence, 3,000 of the animals

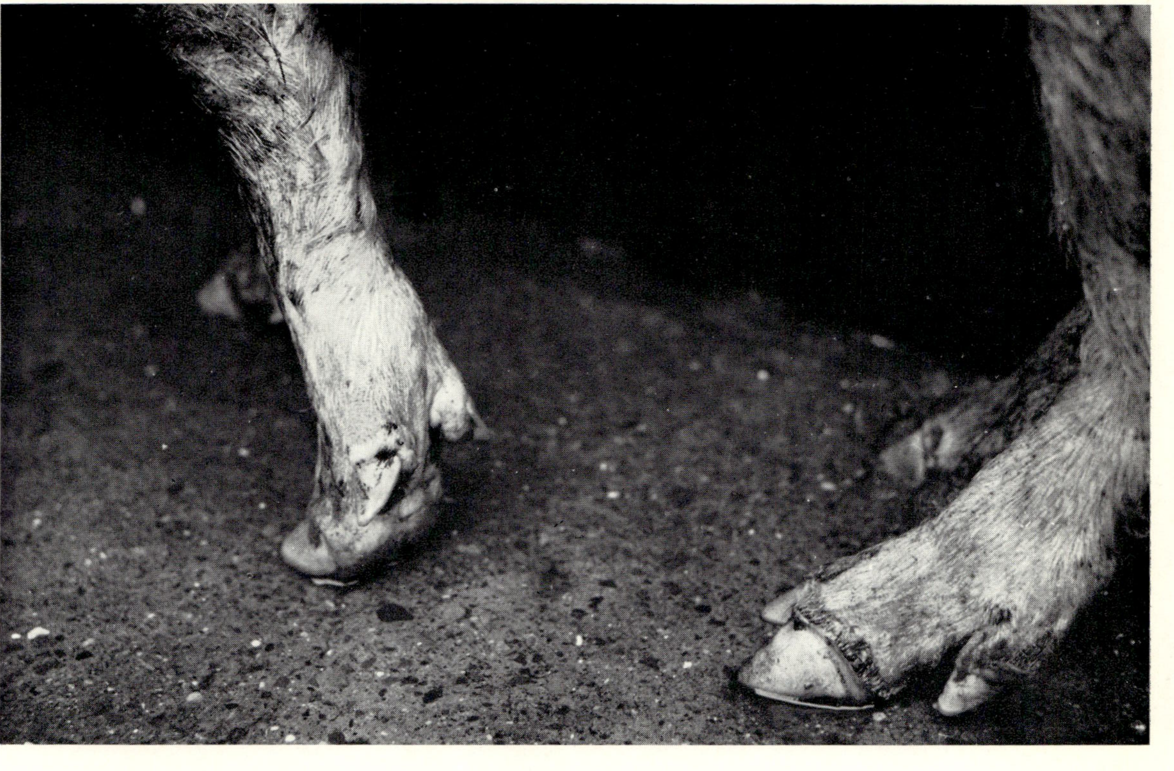

1. Foot and mouth disease in pig vesicles around the coronary band.

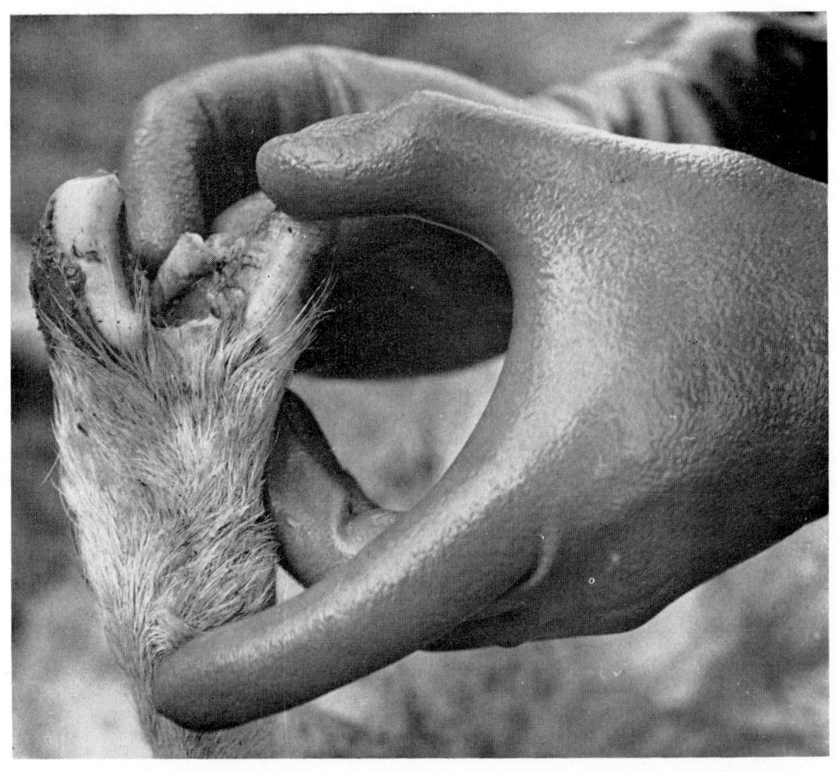

2. Ruptured vesicle in the forefoot of a sheep.   Taken after the
humane slaughter of the animal.   *Crown Copyright*

sold there that day were still on the premises. They were the responsibility of their new owners, who had just bought them by auction, and they could not be taken beyond the 10-mile limit of the infected area. If, therefore, a purchaser happened to live outside that sinister circle, he could either find a farmer within it who was willing to take the animals till the restrictions were lifted or he could have them slaughtered at the nearest abattoir. For most buyers there was no choice. The beasts went direct to the slaughterhouse.

Three topics exercised the minds of northern farmers in these early days. They were worried about (*a*) compensation, (*b*) how the disease was being spread, and (*c*) the secondary effects of the epidemic.

Anxiety on the first score concerned the animals sent straight from Oswestry market to the abattoir. As these were not official "contact" animals but only stock that had to be slaughtered because there was nowhere to keep them, they were not eligible for compensation. The unfortunate purchasers found themselves receiving less than half the price they had just paid, for instance, for a good dairy cow, for such an animal is worth not nearly as much dead as alive. There were, however, comparatively few subsequent complaints about compensation, except that rising values made it necessary to make some adjustments to amounts paid for the earliest victims.

On the spread of the disease, the familiar arguments about starlings, gulls and foxes were soon in full circulation. Of the 40 outbreaks reported to November 2nd, 23 were in Shropshire, within easy distance of Llanyblodwell, and so were presumably connected with the primary outbreak. The subsequent pattern of cases indicated that the infection could well have been wind-borne, for they occurred in a widening arc to the north-east of

Llanyblodwell, at a time when the prevailing wind was, as usual, in the south-west.

It proved impossible to trace any connection between the Shropshire outbreaks and many of those farther afield. As for the primary outbreak, it was not until months later that the Ministry issued a cautious opinion about its cause. As early as November 3rd, however, it pointed out that birds could not have been responsible for the introduction of the disease to Britain. No epidemic was in progress in Holland, Belgium, France or any other countries from which migrating birds come.

The secondary effects quickly promised to be as important as the actual slaughter. The epidemic could hardly have come at a worse time, for the movement of store stock from farm to farm was at its height. Autumn-calving cows and heifers were being transferred from rearing farms to dairies for the winter milking. Their calves, at their most numerous at this time of the year, were being shipped in large numbers to rearing and fattening units. So were store lambs and pigs. As the cows calved, demand for artificial insemination services were at their peak, and these too were summarily stopped. Sheep farmers were unable to bring in rams for the tupping season.

All over the North, agricultural events were cancelled. Among them in the first week of November were the National Agricultural Centre's Open Day at Stoneleigh, the British Friesian Show and Sale at York, and two Milk Marketing Board bulk milk collection demonstrations. Climbers and ramblers were asked to keep away from Snowdonia, where large numbers of sheep roam free.

The Week Ending November 14th

In the second week of November the epidemic escalated, to use a fashionable word of the moment. It raged, in fact, like a forest fire. On November 14th the Minister of Agriculture stated in the House of Commons that the number of outbreaks had reached 330. Approximately 28,000 cattle, 16,000 sheep and 18,000 pigs had been slaughtered, and new cases were being confirmed almost hourly. Over 300 veterinary officers were now at work on the epidemic, including 30 rushed in from Ireland. Although most of the outbreaks were confined to Shropshire, Flintshire, Cheshire, Denbighshire and Montgomeryshire, there had been four cases in Lancashire, two in Staffordshire, two in Derbyshire and one in Westmoreland. The controlled area now extended into Lincolnshire, Leicestershire, Nottinghamshire, Rutland, Huntingdonshire and Warwickshire.

Said Mr Ernest Corrigall, regional veterinary officer for the West Midlands, who was in charge of operations at the headquarters at Oswestry, "In the annals of the Ministry I don't think there have ever been so many outbreaks concentrated into such a comparatively small area in such a small space of time."

Troops were now brought in to help with the disinfecting and cleaning up of infected farms. Several hundreds of slaughtermen were permanently engaged, and more than 25 giant excavators found full employment in digging pits for the burial of slaughtered animals.

The Northern Livestock Show and the livestock classes at the Birmingham Fatstock Show were cancelled, and on November 14th, after much heart-searching, the Royal Smithfield Show, due to be held on December 4th to 8th, also cancelled its livestock classes. All northern meetings likely to attract farmers had, of course, been scrubbed.

Among the early casualties was the export trade in livestock and meat to Europe. This had been building up very satisfactorily during the year, and in particular a lively trade in calves, chiefly to Belgium, had developed during the autumn. All now came to a dead stop. Northern Ireland then banned the import of raw vegetables and potatoes from Great Britain.

It was not to be expected that outstanding flocks and herds would in any way escape the general devastation. Among the early victims was Mr John Atkins, of Bayston Hill, in Shropshire, whose 114-strong Aldbourne herd of British Friesians had taken him seventeen years to build up. Mr Norman Hughes, of Trefowen, near Oswestry, saw his world-famous flock of pedigree Border Leicester sheep destroyed. Mr Geoffrey Dean, of Haughton Hall, Tarporley, Cheshire, lost a prize-winning pedigree herd of 42 Jerseys. The well-known Cheshire cheese-maker, Mr William Wild, of Mollington, Cheshire, had 60 cattle and over 1,000 pigs slaughtered on one of his farms.

Already the compensation total was creeping up towards the £2 million mark, reached by the 1952 epidemic, and farmers were wondering whether it would surpass even that visitation. Had they but known it, their troubles were only beginning.

The Week Ending November 21st

The following week proved the worst for over 40 years. Over 38,000 head of cattle alone were slaughtered, plus nearly 20,000 pigs and over 16,000 sheep. Outbreaks were occurring in such quick succession that it was almost impossible to keep an accurate tally of their numbers, though on the day November 20th the official figure was 639.

The protagonists of the theory that the infection was wind-borne were given confirmation of their ideas when, on November 16th, the wind veered to the north after blowing for a fortnight from the south-west. Almost immediately an outbreak occurred at Spetchley in Worcestershire, an area previously free and lying south of the stricken counties. Next day a further outbreak at Stanway took the disease over the county border into Gloucestershire. The wind-borne theory, however, hardly accounted for new outbreaks in Lancashire. In Derbyshire, Leicestershire, Staffordshire and Montgomeryshire the disease extended its hold systematically, while in Cheshire, Shropshire, Flintshire and Denbighshire it raged unabated. By November 20th the total number of outbreaks in Cheshire had risen to 291 and in Shropshire to 223.

On November 18th the whole of England and Wales was declared a controlled area, the effect being to prohibit the movement of animals throughout the whole country, except under licence. Another order banned the use of unpasteurised milk, skimmed milk and whey for stock food except on the farm of origin, as it was thought that the disease could be spread by these agents.

Cancellations of public events became wholesale. They included the annual general meeting of the Shropshire and West Midlands Agricultural Society and of the Jersey Cattle Society. Also the B.O.C.M. dairy conference at Tunbridge Wells, the Scottish Fatstock Show, the Hereford bull sale, the Galloway Society's autumn show and sale, the Border Friesian bull show and sale, the English Guernsey Cattle Society's autumn show and sale at Reading, and all meetings of the Pig Industry Development Authority. Mr Fred Peart, the Minister of Agriculture, cancelled a visit he was to have made to Pakistan, in order to be on hand to deal with further problems. In the infected areas the Royal Automobile Club cancelled a rally, the Coventry Angling Association called off all fishing, and various hunts, football matches and cycling meetings were crossed off.

Livestock export trade received some further blows. On

December 11th a consignment of 410 Herefords and 50 Aberdeen-Angus cattle, worth £124,600, were due to be shipped to Russia, but now the Russians called off the deal, until six months after Britain became clear of foot-and-mouth disease. Large export orders of Large White pigs to Spain and France were also held up.

Among the more notable victims this week was the West Felton Golden Guernsey herd, of 120 animals, belonging to Mr Hugh Richards, of Sandford Hall, near Oswestry, who also lost 300 other cattle as well as a flock of sheep. Lord Rock-savage saw his herd of 53 Galloways slaughtered at Cholmond-eley Castle, Cheshire. And Messrs T. L. D. Everall & Son lost 79 pedigree Herefords, of the Shradon herd and worth £23,000, at Montford Bridge, Shrewsbury.

Although all northern store markets were closed, the Scottish markets remained open, and special licences from the Ministry enabled some northern farmers to bring down store cattle from Scotland. Some Irish cattle found their way on to northern farms by this route. In general, however, the problems created by the standstill order remained and were intensified. The Milk Marketing Board announced plans for issuing "do-it-yourself" A.I. kits for farmers whom the inseminators were unable to visit. The idea was for the kit to be left at the farm gate and for the farmer to receive instructions by telephone for using it.

The Week Ending November 28th

The fourth week of November proved the worst to date. In the House of Commons on November 27th the Minister of Agriculture gave the total number of outbreaks as 1,156 and the total number of animals slaughtered as 205,000. The latter comprised 102,000 cattle, 43,000 sheep and 60,000 pigs. Mr Peart himself visited the worst plague centres, at Oswestry, Chester and Crewe, on the 24th, when he announced that he would be setting up bureaux to advise farmers on re-stocking later on. On the same day Scotland was declared a controlled area.

The epidemic was now extending its range as well as in its intensity. New outbreaks occurred in Northamptonshire, Gloucestershire and Herefordshire, and infected areas now took in parts of Buckinghamshire and Monmouthshire.

This was indeed a black week for Britain, for it also saw the devaluation of the pound. Farmers' leaders felt exasperated and frustrated that this unique opportunity to step up exports should be nullified by the foot-and-mouth epidemic. Under the circumstances even more restrictions were placed on our overseas trade. The country lived in a state of siege. Northern Ireland prohibited imports of used farm machinery from any part of Great Britain, and Eire imposed severe restrictions on trade and travel across the Irish Sea.

Since the epidemic began opinion among farmers had been hardening against the imports of meat from Argentina, which was strongly suspected of having been responsible for the primary outbreak. Mr Gwilym Williams, president of the National Farmers' Union, now demanded that the import of meat from all countries in which foot-and-mouth disease was endemic should be banned without delay. Mr T. Myrddin Evans, president of the Farmers Union of Wales, made a similar strong protest. Said Mr Gwilym Williams:

"The present outbreak of foot-and-mouth disease has meant breaking delivery dates on a whole range of livestock, both pedigree and commercial. Although our overseas customers have, in the main, been sympathetic, this situation does not make for confidence and long-term business, and costs the country millions of pounds in lost orders. Many previous outbreaks in this country have been traced back to infected imported meat, and it is our view that, if we are to succeed in our export drive, the Government must give our pedigree and commercial livestock producers protection."

Although this demand met with no immediate response the dangers inherent in meat products were underlined by a Ministry notice of November 27th which reminded swill feeders that "they are required by law to keep animals from having contact with unboiled meat, bones, offal or any other part of a carcase of any animal, or with any other waste food which has been in contact with such products. In addition, all waste food must be boiled for at least one hour before it is fed to animals."

Oddly enough, in this week Argentina voluntarily stopped shipments of meat to Britain on the grounds that prices were inadequate. As the epidemic, combined with a dock strike, had been causing a serious shortage of meat in many towns and had driven prices up by as much as 15 per cent, this explanation was difficult to understand.

It was not the only contradictory statement flyng around. The Royal Smithfield Show, having cancelled its livestock classes, was under pressure to close down entirely. This it naturally did not want to do, having regard to the fact that it is the main shop-window of our huge and flourishing export trade in agricultural machinery. In the event, it resisted pressure and held a satisfactory show, without any unfortunate after-effects. When the decision was still in the balance, however, the Minister of Agriculture told the House of Commons "that there has been no evidence of mechanical transfer (of the virus) by human movement or vehicles", a statement which the Smithfield Show Council must have felt highly encouraging though hardly credible.

Down in the infected areas, however, Ministry officials were still busy disinfecting tyres and boots. Farmers were urged not to organise or attend shoots. All race meetings were cancelled, and horses from infected areas were banned from the Newmarket bloodstock sales. Representatives of firms selling goods to farmers were confined to their offices, whence they transacted business by telephone. The Irish Government banned the entry of all motor vehicles from Britain to Irish ports and begged its nationals to stay away. The Potato Marketing Board cancelled its annual general meeting, and the National Poultry Show, which normally coincides with the last days of the Smithfield Show and is also held in London, was likewise closed.

Anxiety was felt for the sheep ranging over the Pennines from Derbyshire northwards. Hill farmers were glad to get their flocks off the fells for tupping, and most of them decided to keep them penned while the epidemic lasted. Down in the New Forest, too, the rounding-up of the free-ranging cattle and pigs began.

The slaughter bill was now assuming such alarming proportions that alternatives to the slaughter policy were widely debated by press and public. The pros and cons of vaccination were thoroughly aired, and Mr H. Pakenham Hamilton, the Duke of Westminster's herd manager in 1923, issued a pamphlet describing how he helped to cure a foot-and-mouth disease outbreak on the Duke's Eaton Hall estate in that year. While opinion in general continued to support the slaughter policy, the Minister of Agriculture, in a written reply in the House of Commons on November 28th, announced that, purely as a precaution, he had "arranged for a sufficient supply of vaccine to be acquired and stored in this country to enable a vaccination programme to be adopted as a second line of defence, should this become inevitable".

The Week Ending December 5th

So to the end of November and the first week of December, when the epidemic showed the first signs of being past its peak. The number of outbreaks per day fell from around 70 to the 30s, and the total of cattle slaughtered in the week ending December 5th fell from near 43,000 in the previous week to about 25,000. Disastrous enough, in all truth, yet still an improvement. The disease was reported from no new counties this week, but the controlled areas were extended in several counties, notably in Lancashire and Leicestershire.

On December 1st, Mr Peart announced to the House of Commons a ban on meat imports from all but a few countries "where the disease was unknown or which had a long history of freedom from it". A Parliamentary debate on the epidemic generated a lot of heat but provided little extra illumination on matters of fact or policy.

Chief criticism levelled against the Minister concerned lack of determination and uniformity in dealing with public events and with advice on disinfectants. The holding of Smithfield Show when so many other meetings were banned was still a lively topic, and Members of Parliament gave instances of angling contests and similar events in infected areas.

With regard to disinfectants, somewhat conflicting and confusing statements did little to help the situation and played into the hands of the old Cheshire farmer who swore that disinfectants were helping to spread the disease! Inquirers were advised, at various times, by Ministry officials (*a*) to use any of the disinfectants listed under the Diseases of Animals Order (nearly 300 of them), (*b*) to keep off coal tar derivatives unless they contained at least 1 per cent hexachlorophene, (*c*) that a solution of washing soda was best, and (*d*) not to use washing soda where it would come into contact with metal, paintwork or fabric. The National Farmers' Union eventually sorted out the recommendations to the extent of advising that washing soda solution was probably best for "rubber boots, utensils and woodwork", hypochlorite solutions for human and animal skin, and carbolic disinfectants for floors and roads. It added, however, that "any disinfectant is, as a general rule, better than none".

Meanwhile, as we shall see from the testimony of some of the victims in a later chapter, some farms which observed every possible precaution nevertheless caught the disease. There was also doubt about the efficacy or otherwise of barriers of straw soaked in disinfectant placed across roads. Such barriers were constructed, and manned by relays of volunteers, as far south as Devonshire, but the Ministry expressed doubts as to whether they achieved anything. They advocated instead similar barriers at the entrances to farms. Yet on November 28th barriers on road bridges across the Thames were manned by soldiers from army units which had been instructed that such precautions were to take priority over all training exercises.

The Irish Minister of Agriculture, Mr Neil T. Blaney, declared that he was horrified to think that "one careless person could bring the disease to Ireland and cause havoc having the dimensions of a national disaster". As Irish exports of livestock and livestock products total about £112 million a year, he was not exaggerating. He appealed to all Irishmen planning to return home to visit their families at Christmas to stay where they were. If they felt they must come from Britain, they were (*a*) to travel light and bring only recently laundered clothing, (*b*) to fill in conscientiously an entry card and to report on arrival to the Ministry of Agriculture, and (*c*) to stay away from all livestock on farms.

Insurance cover for consequential loss from foot-and-mouth disease became very expensive and difficult to obtain. Lloyds' underwriters found it impossible to get cover for any farm within 50 miles of an outbreak, while rates charged outside such a radius rose to £5 per head for cattle, as against half-a-crown before the epidemic.

In spite of the general approval of the Minister's ban on meat imports, some of the beef breed societies were anxious about its effects on them. The South American countries are among their best customers, and they worried about reprisals.

By the end of the week nearly 700 veterinary officers, including some from Australia, Canada and New Zealand, were fighting the epidemic. But on December 4th the number of outbreaks took an alarming upward swing, to 58 for the day. For December 5th it was 53.

At a press conference at Crewe on December 5th the Cheshire county branch of the National Farmers' Union stated that over half of the outbreaks to date (763 out of a total of 1,508 for the whole country) had occurred in Cheshire. The county had lost 65,085 cattle, 11,690 sheep and 31,752 pigs, and the epidemic had cut down the production of Cheshire cheese by 25 per cent.

The Week Ending December 12th

In the second week of December (to December 12th) a further fall in the number of outbreaks occurred, and this steady decline continued till the epidemic finally ended. Outbreaks were still occurring at an alarming level, however, nearly 19,000 head of stock being slaughtered during the week. On December 8th the Oswestry centre confessed to a feeling of "guarded optimism", the number of outbreaks having fallen to 26 on that day, as compared with 47 on the previous day.

On the same day, however, an outbreak in a new district, in Kesteven, Lincolnshire, 50 miles from the nearest infected area, caused fresh anxiety. This was on the farm of North Hykeham, near Lincoln. At first there were fears that it might have been caused not by the virus responsible for the other outbreaks but by an even more violent and devastating virus which had made its appearance in three of the westernmost republics of the Soviet Union. Dr J. B. Brooksby, director of the Animal Virus Research Unit at Pirbright, Surrey, warned that if this eastern virus, the A–22 strain, were to penetrate into Europe it "would make the Cheshire outbreaks look like kids' stuff".

Meat imports were also banned from South Africa because of a new outbreak there.

On December 7th and 8th blizzards swept much of the country, adding to the hardships of the infected regions. The Ministry of Agriculture became particularly concerned about the situation in the Peak District National Park. Snow, and the imminence of Christmas which tempted motorists into the countryside to collect holly and other greenery, coincided with several foot-and-mouth outbreaks around Bakewell, and the danger to flocks of sheep on the open moorland became desperate. The Ministry's appeal to visitors to keep away met, on the whole, with a satisfactory response.

On the credit side, a reduction of the controlled area in Monmouthshire allowed the Severn Bridge to be re-opened to livestock transport. And the Ministry made a welcome announcement of a special ploughing-up grant of £10 an acre to assist farmers who had lost livestock through the disease.

Overseas, the Argentine Government quickly reacted to our ban on the import of Argentine meat by prohibiting its buyers from attending the December bloodstock sales at Newmarket. The prohibition, stated to be a deliberate reprisal, cost the bloodstock industry at least a million dollars. Irish breeders and buyers were, of course, absent from the sales, and the Japanese stayed away too. Eire continued to take the epidemic extremely seriously, and Dublin Zoo was closed for the first time since the 1916 Easter Rising. The Irish Government deplored the fact that British Railways were still inviting traffic to Ireland under special Christmas terms, in spite of Irish appeals to would-be visitors to stay away.

At home, it was decided to cancel the popular Oxford Farming Conference, due to be held on January 8th to 10th. And the racing authorities continued to fight a losing battle for Boxing Day racing fixtures.

France banned all racehorses and other animals from Britain, and New Zealand prohibited the import of all British agricultural and horticultural products.

As the epidemic abated the criticisms of the handling of almost every aspect of it increased. In Cheshire a group of about twenty farmers who had lost their stock in the epidemic but whose farms were now free from infection met to form a Cheshire Farmers' Club. The Chairman was Mr Reg Roberts, of The Old Farm, Barrow, near Chester, and one of the first objectives of the Club was to plan for the re-stocking of the stricken farms.

The Week Ending December 19th

In the week to December 19th there was a further decrease in the number of outbreaks, the total number of cattle slaughtered being just short of 15,000. On December 19th the number of outbreaks for the day fell to 17, the lowest for six weeks. The whole of Monmouthshire was declared free, and the infected area boundaries were narrowed in Warwickshire, Worcestershire and Gloucestershire. Setbacks occurred, however. A few hours after restrictions were eased around Bosbury, in Herefordshire, a new outbreak caused them to be imposed again. New outbreaks in the Lincolnshire village of South Hykeham, where the original Lincolnshire outbreak occurred, resulted in the entire livestock population of the village being destroyed.

With the approach of Christmas, with the accompanying increase in travel and sporting events, further restrictions were announced. The Ministry of Agriculture advised against the holding of football matches on or near farmland anywhere near infected areas and asked that people from infected areas should not attend sporting events outside. The New Zealand All Blacks, completing their rugby tour on the 16th, had every bit of clothing dry-cleaned and their kit washed in disinfectant.

The presidents of the Country Landowners' Association and of the National Farmers' Union added their appeals to those of the Minister that all organised shoots over farmland anywhere in the country should stop. The Minister banned shooting parties in infected areas or in any county adjoining an infected area.

The Chief Scout, Sir Charles Maclean, told scouts to keep within their own areas for outdoor activities, and London scouts in particular were asked to postpone visits to the country. In the Lake District the Youth Hostels Association closed its thirty hostels till January 11th, cancelling 500 Christmas bookings.

Ireland stepped up her restrictions by announcing that anyone from Britain visiting an Irish farm within twenty-one days of arriving in Ireland would be liable to a fine of £100 or two months' imprisonment. A man who arrived in Dublin on the 14th, after allegedly passing through foot-and-mouth infected areas in England, was ordered not to leave the city for 21 days. From midnight on December 13th British Railways stopped issuing tickets to Ireland. All arrangements to run special services to Ireland for Christmas were cancelled. Shipowners, especially those trading with Ireland and South America, complained that their trade was being very seriously hit.

The Ministry of Agriculture issued advice to people leaving an infected area to holiday at home for Christmas. Having pointed out that anyone living on an infected farm could leave only with the written consent of the veterinary officer in charge, it gave the following instructions for those resident on un-infected farms in infected areas:

"(*a*) avoid coming into contact with any farm animal or going into fields or places where there are animals or where animals may be driven later;

(*b*) disinfect all footwear to be used;

(*c*) wear clothes which have had no possible contact with farm animals. If there is any doubt, clothes should be dry-cleaned;

(*d*) wash with plenty of hot water and soap, not forgetting the hair;

(*e*) disinfect the outside of any suitcase that may have been in contact with other articles in general use on the farm."

Japan announced on the 12th a ban on all livestock imports from Britain and said that a strict medical check would be conducted on all passengers from Britain.

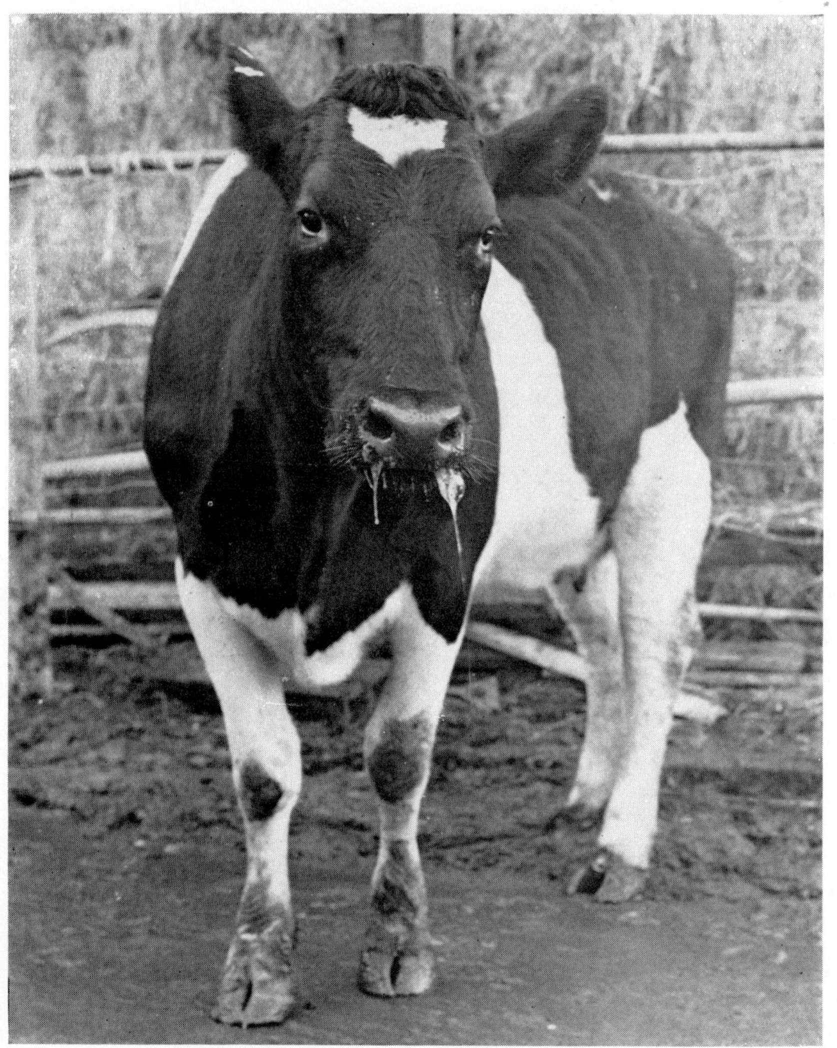

3. Friesian Cow showing salivation due to foot and mouth disease.

Crown Copyright

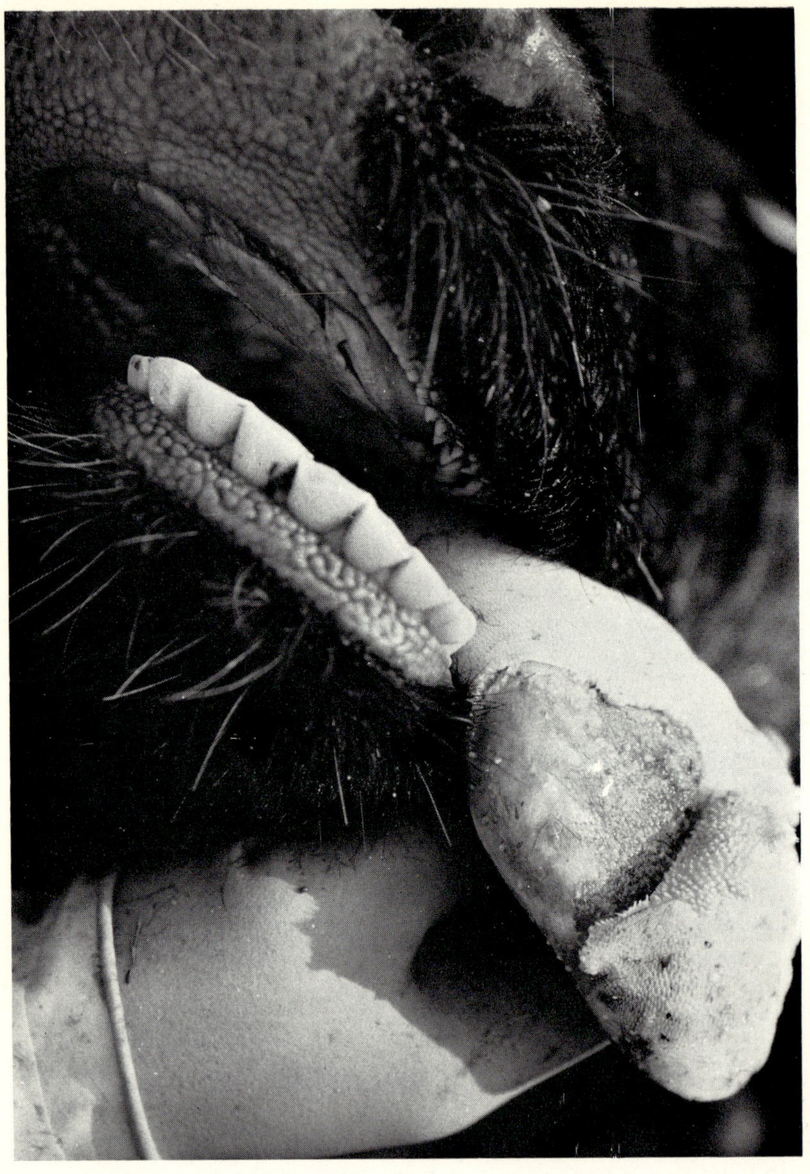

4. Ruptured vesicle on tongue of cow. Taken after the humane slaughter of the animal.

Crown Copyright

The annual general meeting of the National Farmers' Union, due to have been held in London on January 22nd to 24th, was postponed.

The National Farmers' Union announced a plan to compile a register of all farmers willing to make stock available for sale to those who had lost their flocks and herds.

On December 17th the Irish Government took half-page advertisements in the British Press, advising visitors to stay away and warning of strict penalties and long delays. There is, too, they said, a total ban on imports of meat, meat products, vegetables and other agricultural products, and "all parcels from Britain which contain or include clothing or used foot-wear will be automatically returned to sender. THIS IS A NATIONAL EMERGENCY."

Over the same week-end British Railways announced that, from Monday, December 18th, all sailings of their boats from Holyhead and Fishguard would be cancelled. It also banned the sale of tickets to Northern Ireland though this ban was soon modified to allow sailings from northern ports. British European Airways cancelled 60 per cent of its Christmas bookings. Aer Lingus cut its bookings by 75 per cent.

One of the worst outbreaks of the week occurred at the Kesteven College of Agriculture at Caythorpe, near Lincoln, where nearly 600 pedigree cattle and pigs and a flock of 250 sheep, worth in all £25,000, were slaughtered.

The Week of Christmas

Christmas in the stricken areas was, naturally, a grim affair, relieved only by the continuing evidence that the epidemic was abating. In the week to December 26th, the number of animals killed fell to just over 21,000, of which over 4,000 were in Cheshire, which county had 34 outbreaks.

Infected areas were reduced in size in Worcestershire and Warwickshire, but new outbreaks extended the infected areas in Derbyshire and Nottinghamshire. A new outbreak among sheep at Penkridge, in Staffordshire, aroused concern for the safety of deer in Cannock Chase, since they were susceptible to the disease and could act as carriers. The 24 cases reported on December 20th brought the total number of outbreaks in the epidemic to 2,001.

The Week Ending January 2nd, 1968

By January 2nd, 1968, the average daily number of outbreaks had dropped to 13. The infected area was now steadily contracting in many districts, including south Lancashire, Northamptonshire, Rutland, Huntingdonshire and Peterborough. The situation was also improving in Cheshire and Shropshire, but Staffordshire and Derbyshire were reporting many new outbreaks, and one in Nottinghamshire extended the infected area there. Relaxation of movement restriction outside the infected areas allowed store calves and pigs to be widely distributed. An outbreak on December 31st among sheep in an area of Denbighshire around Llangollen densely populated by sheep flocks caused considerable anxiety. Infected area restrictions were removed from much of south Herefordshire, and over in Norfolk the lifting of the ban on shooting enabled a shoot to be held at Sandringham on New Year's Day.

The National Federation of Meat Traders warned the Minister of Agriculture that beef prices would climb to record heights if the ban on importing Argentine meat continued. Fishing-tackle manufacturers estimated they were losing £100,000 a week through lost trade.

Irish farmers were invited to contribute to a calf pool from which British farms would be re-stocked.

Dissatisfaction over the valuation of slaughtered stock continued to rise.

The Week Ending January 9th

In the second week of January the number of outbreaks per day continued to fall. By January 6th it was down to six, and on the 8th it was only two. The number of animals slaughtered in this week was less than 4,000. On January 6th a scare arose from the occurrence of a suspected outbreak on the Isle of Sheppey, in Kent, but tests proved negative.

Further reductions occurred in the infected areas of Lancashire, Yorkshire and Lincolnshire, and even in Cheshire a few parishes were declared clear. Eight race-courses were re-opened, as the ban on racing was eased. It was estimated that this ban which had lasted from November 25th, 1967, to January 5th, 1968, cost the Exchequer over £1½ million in lost gambling tax. The betting turnover was down by an estimated £60 million.

After being closed to climbers and ramblers for two months the Lake District was re-opened.

On January 3rd one of the first farmers to lose his stock in the epidemic began to re-stock. He was Mr Clive Rymond, of Benn Hills Farm, Sheepy Magna, Leicestershire, who lost his Friesian herd on November 19th.

The National Farmers' Union completed its plan to create a register of stock available for sale to farmers who had lost their animals in the epidemic. Several of the cattle breed societies were also preparing their own schemes.

On January 8th, Royal Air Force men who had been helping to fight the disease were withdrawn, since it was felt that civilian workers could now cope. In all, nearly 1,900 R.A.F. men had been engaged in the campaign.

The Week Ending January 16th

In the third week of January the epidemic was obviously dying away. Only one case per day occurred on the 18th and 19th. On the other hand, the discovery of the disease in a slaughter-house at Newthorpe, Nottinghamshire, on January 9th caused great alarm. The animals concerned had come from a farm at Sandiacre and had passed through Nottingham market. Ministry officials had the task of tracing all other animals that had passed through the market.

In Herefordshire and Radnorshire farmers were warned by the Ministry not to feed kale to their cattle. It was thought that the crop might have been contaminated by birds from infected areas. Moves to re-open the markets at Ledbury and Ross-on-Wye were postponed after protests by farmers that this was premature. Although Hereford market was re-opened, auctioneers agreed not to sell cattle there for at least two weeks, "in the interests of all farmers".

On January 14th the disease jumped to a new area when it struck a farm at Great Oxenden, in Northamptonshire. This outbreak caused considerable alarm for the safety of the rare deer which roam the Duke of Bedford's park at Woburn, not far away. A suspected case at Hillingdon, Middlesex, fortunately proved negative.

Experts visiting Britain from the Argentina declared that the foot-and-mouth disease virus, O_1, which was responsible for the epidemic is of European origin and could not be blamed on Argentinian meat. The Ministry of Agriculture experts were not convinced.

Interest this week centred largely on schemes for re-stocking, which were now gathering momentum. They were given impetus by Her Majesty the Queen who on January 10th sent the following message to the Minister of Agriculture:

"I have been greatly concerned by the extent and severity of the present epidemic of foot-and-mouth disease.

I wish to express my deep sympathy for the farmers who have so tragically lost their livestock and my admiration for all who have been fighting with such untiring efforts to control the disease and to rid the country of it once again.

When you have succeeded in this there will begin the formidable task of re-stocking the stricken farms. This will be eased by the help you are giving.

I understand that there is a scheme for those farmers who, at the end of the present epidemic, find themselves unaffected, to be able to help those who have lost all their animals.

I wholeheartedly support this effort and when the time is right I wish to contribute to this pool of livestock from the Royal farms. I am sure that this scheme will appeal to a very large number of farmers."

The Week Ending January 23rd

In the fourth week of January, life was returning to normal in the countryside over much of England and Wales. Sports events, shooting and fishing were resumed (though not, of course, in infected areas), and on January 22nd the first auction market for farm animals anywhere in England and Wales since November 17th was held at Aberystwyth.

Small numbers of outbreaks, however, continued to occur, and one of them was on a farm at Laxton, Nottinghamshire, occupied by Mr John Rose as bailiff for Mr Fred Peart, Minister of Agriculture, who is Lord of the Manor there. One effect of this outbreak was again to put a long stretch of the A1 road out of bounds to livestock transport, compelling motor vehicles carrying cattle, sheep and pigs to make a long detour.

The National Farmers' Union expressed concern about the abundance of foxes in many hill districts, following the ban on hunting throughout the winter. Fears were felt for the safety of lambs when the lambing season began.

The Ministry of Agriculture announced that advisory centres had been set up in the infected areas, to help farmers with problems that arose when their farms were declared free. It was estimated that Cheshire, Shropshire and Staffordshire alone had lost 137,000 dairy cattle.

The Week Ending January 30th

In the fourth and last week of January outbreaks dropped to about one a day, though with occasional relapses. (There were, for instance, five cases on the 24th.) The 27th was the first clear day since the epidemic began on October 25th.

From midnight on January 30th the whole of Scotland, together with Cumberland and Northumberland, ceased to be a controlled area.

The Minister of Agriculture made an Order, as from January 26th, prohibiting the release from storage of all imported meat from countries in the suspension of imports, and which had been in store before the ban had been imposed.

The temporary ban on imports from countries in which foot-and-mouth disease is endemic was made on December 4th for three months. On January 24th, Mr John Mackie, joint parliamentary secretary to the Ministry of Agriculture, refused in the House of Commons to give an undertaking that the ban would be extended until an independent inquiry into the epidemic, which was shortly to be set up, had issued its report. A row blew up in consequence, and Mr Gwilym Williams, president of the National Farmers' Union, sent a strong protest to the Minister.

The Week Ending February 6th

The first week of February saw outbreaks occurring at the rate of one or two a day, all in existing infected areas. Two on February 5th brought the total for the epidemic to 2,325.

Pressure on the Minister to retain the ban on imported meat increased.

Within the first week after the nation-wide distribution of forms by the National Farmers' Union inviting assistance with re-stocking plans for stricken farms, offers of more than 22,000 cattle and 17,000 sheep had been received. The Royal Agricultural Benevolent Institution made available the sum of £4,000 to help farming families who had experienced severe hardship as a result of the epidemic. It also kept open a fund for the purpose, to which farmers and friends could contribute.

Controlled area restrictions were removed from all counties south of the Thames and from East Anglia, some northern counties and parts of South Wales.

The Week Ending February 13th

The week ending February 13th saw a further relaxation of controls. The only areas continuing under controlled area restrictions were the entire counties of Cheshire, Shropshire, Flint, Hereford, Worcester, Stafford, Derby, Lincoln, Nottingham, Leicester, Rutland, Northampton, and Warwick, and parts of Lancashire, the West Riding of Yorkshire, Denbigh, Merioneth, Montgomery, Radnor, Peterborough and Huntingdon—in fact, the areas in which outbreaks had been concentrated. Snowdonia National Park lay in the area thus freed. However, outbreaks still continued to occur, though all in infected areas. There were two, in Derby and Stafford, on the 13th.

In a mounting campaign against the Minister's hesitation about continuing the ban on imported meat from Argentina, the National Federation of Women's Institutes, with over 250,000 members, strongly supported the National Farmers' Union in its fight for the retention of the ban.

The Weeks Ending February 27th

February 17th saw what could have been a very serious setback. Mr F. H. Robinson's Bredicote Court Farm at Spetchley, near Worcester, was the scene of one of the early outbreaks, in November. After the usual complete disinfecting, it was declared free in January, and Mr Robinson set about re-stocking. The first cows were moved in on January 18th. On February 17th one of them was found to be suffering from foot-and-mouth disease in the very early stages. The normal slaughter policy was immediately followed. The infected cow, and most of the others, came from the Swindon district of Wiltshire, well outside any infected area, and it therefore appeared that the infection must have survived on the farm. In his first visitation Mr Robinson lost 230 cows and 400 sheep; in the second outbreak, 80 cows and 130 sheep.

The president of the National Farmers' Union sent a telegram to the Prime Minister asking him to intervene to maintain the ban on imported meat from countries where foot-and-mouth disease is endemic.

The Minister of Agriculture announced that the Duke of Northumberland, who has been chairman of the Agricultural Research Council since 1958, was to be chairman of the committee of inquiry into the Ministry's policy for dealing with foot-and-mouth disease.

Within the following week, two further outbreaks occurred on farms which had already been cleared after the first outbreak.

The Ministry pointed out that these three cases were the only ones from 182 farms which had been re-stocked. It nevertheless announced a new set of safeguards, primarily a series of inspections, to be applied to re-stocked farms.

The End of Epidemic

So we come to March 4th, when Mr Peart, who had been subjected to severe pressure from all sides to make an announcement on the origin of the epidemic and on the future of the ban on imported meat, reported to the House of Commons. The Minister based his decisions on the report of his chief veterinary officer, Mr John Reid, who summarised his conclusions as follows:

"1. I have been unable to discover any possible source of the infection except Argentine lamb.

2. Although there is not conclusive evidence that Argentine lamb was the source, I am of the opinion that there is sufficient circumstantial evidence for concluding that this lamb was the cause of the initial case on Bryn Farm and some of the other cases."

Thus fortified, Mr Peart announced a political compromise of classic character. The ban on imports of mutton and lamb from countries where foot-and-mouth disease is endemic would, he said, be continued for the time being; but the ban on imported beef would be lifted on April 15th.

Farmers, landowners and their allies leapt to protest. Mr Gwilym Williams, president of the National Farmers' Union, called the decision "a cynical and arbitrary device". The Country Landowners' Association dubbed it "a compromise and not a logical decision". At the time of writing the controversy grows fiercer and looks like engaging agricultural attention for some time.

Meantime, with epidemic conditions finally petering out in late February, the final totals of animals slaughtered were: cattle 208,811; sheep 100,699; pigs 113,423. The percentages of the total flocks and herds in England and Wales were: for cattle, 2·5 per cent; for sheep, 0·54 per cent; for pigs, 2·06 per cent.

In the stricken counties, however, the ratios were much higher. Cheshire lost 33·1 per cent of its cattle, 33 per cent of its pigs, and 16·3 per cent of its sheep. Shropshire, 19·1 per cent of its cattle, 23·4 per cent of its pigs and 6·06 per cent of its sheep. Flintshire, 17·5 per cent of its cattle, 31·7 per cent of its pigs, and 5·6 per cent of its sheep. Denbighshire, 6·1 per cent of its cattle, 10·6 per cent of its pigs, and 0·9 per cent of its sheep.

The total cost of the epidemic is reckoned to be in excess of £100 million, of which £35 million will be the cost to the Exchequer, paid in compensation for slaughtered animals.

Last Kick

In early March, when the epidemic seemed to be in its last throes, it was announced that it would be officially over at 5 p.m. on March 13th. Unhappily, new outbreaks occurred. Not many, but one every now and then, just as everyone was beginning to feel secure. Some of these were on re-stocked farms, a fact which gave rise to widespread alarm. Others were on farms which had hitherto escaped. In April, these sporadic outbreaks were still cropping up, but by the month's end had ceased.

[5]

The Human Victims

Every outbreak is a heartbreak. In the future, when farmers manage their giant estates from an office desk by remote control and computers, cows and sheep may be no more than digits on a page of statistics. For the present, they are still sentient creatures of flesh-and-blood, with personalities and idiosyncracies known well to the farmer and his men.

Farmers' sons and daughters begin their farming career by caring for pet lambs and calves, and they never lose a personal feeling for their stock. The farm children of Cheshire and Shropshire saw their pet lambs and calves sacrificed and had to be reassured that their beloved ponies would not suffer the same fate. The experience was no less harrowing for the farmer himself, who saw the obliteration of a lifetime's work in the slaughter of herds whose ancestors he had carefully selected for four or five generations.

Mr Reg Roberts, of The Old Farm, Barrow, Chester, has described in a letter written to me on December 18th, 1967, how foot-and-mouth disease hit his farms.

"Together with my two sons we farm five farms, situated near to Chester and all adjoining. They are devoted to dairy, pigs and corn, with approximately 260 cows in two herds, 100 breeding sows and 200 acres of barley. We also handle between 6,000 and 7,000 cattle per year, bought on commission for dairy farmers all over the British Isles. We maintain our own herds as nearly self-contained units, this policy being necessary to give our first-class herdsmen an interest in their cows.

I myself always milk at week-ends, partly to relieve one man but also to give me direct contact with my herds. As I am often away all the week, buying cattle, this has been the joy of my life, to get into the parlour and help with the milking.

When the foot-and-mouth disease epidemic broke out in our own county and cases were becoming more numerous every day, we divided the men between the farms and from that time kept strictly to our own farms. No one left the farms, and there were no visitors at all. We took every precaution we could possibly think of.

It was on Saturday morning, November 18th. My stockman and I were milking in the parlour. One cow came in frothing at the mouth and very lame. I knew immediately what it was. We just stared at one another and then both broke down crying. We knew then just how much this was going to change our whole lives. How we finished milking that morning I do not know, but out of sympathy for our cows we just had to do it.

At 8 a.m. we reported it to the Ministry, who sent along a young veterinary surgeon immediately. The disease was confirmed before 9 a.m. The vet immediately started to order materials required to burn the animals, for underground springs forbade disposal of the carcases by burial.

The valuer came at 2 p.m., and this was really a heartbreaking job. My role was to explain to him the qualities of the cattle, with such details as their breeding, milk records, calving dates and brucella tests. To have to talk about what good servants your cows had been, knowing well that within a short time they would all be dead, was an appalling experience. The valuation completed, it was agreed by the valuer, the

Ministry vet and myself, though goodness knows I could not have cared less at that time what value they put on them.

As soon as this was over, the Ministry vet and I decided where the cows were to be shot and where the fire was to be made. At 4 p.m. the slaughtermen arrived. Forty cows were driven into the hayshed and shot. Forty more were then driven in for the same fate. The remainder were driven in on top of them and shot also.

I shall never forget the sound of those guns or the sight of one hundred and forty of the best Friesian cows lying steaming, three deep, in that shed. The calves and young cattle were collected together to meet the same sad end. By the time this job was finished it was 8 p.m., so, not having the materials to start making the fire, we had to fix up lights to keep foxes and vermin from the dead cattle till daybreak.

The numerous outbreaks in Cheshire at this time had caused incendiary materials, and coal in particular, to be in short supply. Although we started to make the pyre on Sunday morning, it took until Wednesday to complete it. We used 450 bales of straw, three lorry-loads of tyres, 200 gallons of oil, 250 railway sleepers and 45 tons of coal.

Because of the lapse of time, the cattle were in an awful mess, and it was a sickening job for the workmen. You can imagine what a gruesome sight the fire was, right in front of our kitchen window. Ninety yards long and twenty feet wide, it burned for three days. The bulldozer then dug a hole, buried the ashes, and levelled off the soil . . . and we were left with our memories. Our farm men were taken over by the Ministry and given instructions to disinfect everything thoroughly. Every shed and yard, every nook and corner, were scrubbed from roof to floor in preparation for the day of re-stocking. . . .

It is very difficult to put into words one's feelings over such a tragedy as this. The silent yards. The empty fields. The despondency of your workers. The look of incomprehension on the sheep-dog's face. You drink a lot, and smoke a lot, and do your best to get a night's sleep. The food nearly chokes you when you go in for meals, and the days seem twice as long as ever they did before.

Since this outbreak we have suffered much the same procedure on four of our other farms. We have only the pig farm left, where my younger son has been a prisoner for six weeks.

We now hear radio programmes we never had time to hear before and we watch television for hours on end, but the one thing we cannot get used to is to go through the day without having a cow to milk, a calf to tend or even an old sow to feed."

In the *Sunday Times* on December 3rd, Jeremy Bugler reported on a visit to Bronington, in Flintshire, in the middle of the epidemic area. He found Mr and Mrs Starkey at the village post office had been taking extraordinary precautions to keep the disease away from their farm behind their house. Mrs Starkey used to wash all the coins she handled in a bowl of disinfectant. She baked letters and newspapers in a hot oven. Wire-netting barriers were erected to keep birds out of the barns, and no crumbs were shaken out from table-cloths. But the Starkey herd went down with the disease, and the post office stood deserted by its former customers.

Social life in the stricken areas came virtually to a standstill. The Women's Institute, the Young Farmers' Club, the National Farmers' Union branch, all ceased to meet. Church attendance dwindled to a handful. Many children stayed away from school, some being sent to relations in distant towns, so that they would miss seeing the distressing sights all around. Even public houses were closed for much of the time.

In Worcestershire five men, engaged by a contractor to assist in burying slaughtered stock, were sacked. Their offence was to leave the farms and visit public-houses at lunch-time.

When the little village of South Hykeham in Lincolnshire was attacked, within about a week every animal in the place had been slaughtered. The losses ranged from over 600 pigs on a large farm to five pigs kept by a farm worker in a cottage sty. Among the casualties were all the animals on a farm purchased in the previous year by Mr Ronald Robinson from a £30,000 pools win. Here the local school was closed, as was the village school at Eaton Constantine, near Shrewsbury. As a safety measure to protect the animals on the school farm of Sleaford Secondary School, in Lincolnshire, the school broke up for the Christmas holidays four days early.

Young Tricia and Edward Nicholas, of Sutton Farm, West Felton, near Oswestry, got their picture into the papers. Their father, Tom Nicholas, lost all his stock in an outbreak on Boxing Day, including the children's pets. Ten-year-old Tricia and six-year-old Edward were sent away so that they should not see the slaughter. Their story so touched the heart of a little girl, eight-year-old Helen Hamersley, who lives on a farm near Perth in Western Australia that she sent them, via the *Daily Mirror*, a cheque for £1 17s. 6d.

Though farmers and their families were the worst sufferers they were not by any means the only people whose lives were disrupted. Not all farm workers were as fortunate as David Hugh and Malcolm MacDonald, who went north to Scotland with their employer when he started up operations there after losing his herd in Cheshire. As described in an earlier chapter, Mr R. C. Hollinshead, of Hoolgrave Manor Farm, Minshull Vernon, near Crewe, lost his herd of 164 Friesians on November 24th. Instead of waiting till restrictions were removed on his own farm, Mr Hollinshead went to Scotland and bought a new Friesian herd, of 112 heifers, from Mr T. C. Bell, of Stravenhouse Farm, Carluke, Lanarkshire. He had to find lodgings for himself and for David Hugh and Malcolm MacDonald while they ran the herd in its old Scottish home, by permission of Mr Bell, but at least he was providing work for his men and an income for himself.

Many farm workers, however, found themselves virtually unemployed. After the slaughter, the Ministry employed the staff of the infected farm for a time, to do the disinfecting and scrubbing down, but then the time of idleness began. Many farms kept on their men, doing such jobs as ditching and draining, but at the basic minimum wage of £10 16s. per week. And these were stockmen who, by working overtime at week-ends, regularly earned much more than the minimum wage. The north-west Midlands, where the epidemic was con-centrated, is a prosperous industrial area, and beyond doubt numbers of farm workers were attracted away from the farms forever, though the total is unknown.

In a way, the farms first stricken by the plague were the lucky ones. They at least knew the worst. For those which escaped to begin with, the tension built up unbearably. For weeks they lived in a state of siege, taking every conceivable precaution but knowing that all their efforts might be in vain. The disease was capricious. It would sweep by them, taking in most of their neighbours in a broad swathe; then, several weeks later, would double back and strike at random a farm here and there that had hitherto escaped. As late as April 1968 farms which had survived in the heart of the infected areas were thus being attacked. There was no security, no peace of mind.

Trade was entirely disrupted. Throughout the whole of

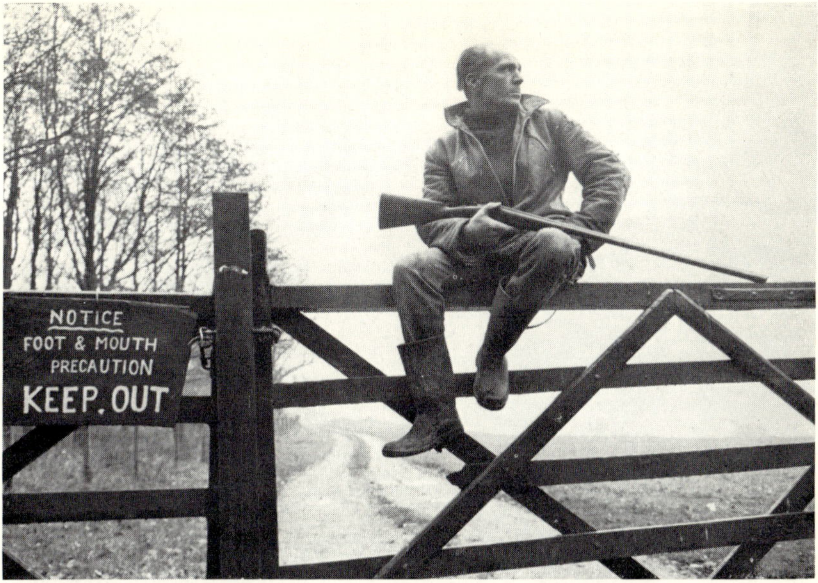

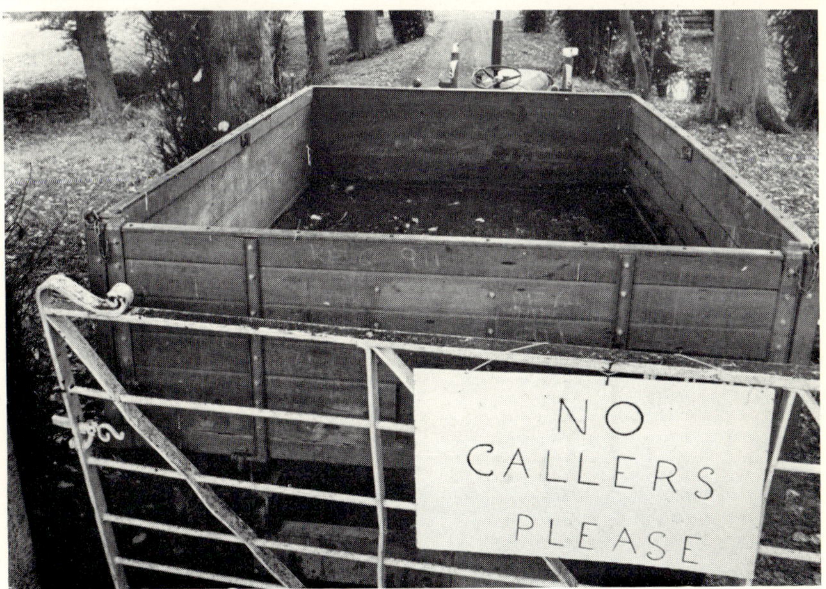

5. *Above:* During the height of the disease inquisitive members of the public were not welcome in affected areas. *The Field*

6. *Below:* A firm but polite keep-out sign on the gate of the Oswestry police station where the Ministry of Agriculture had their headquarters. All movement in affected areas was kept to a minimum. *The Field*

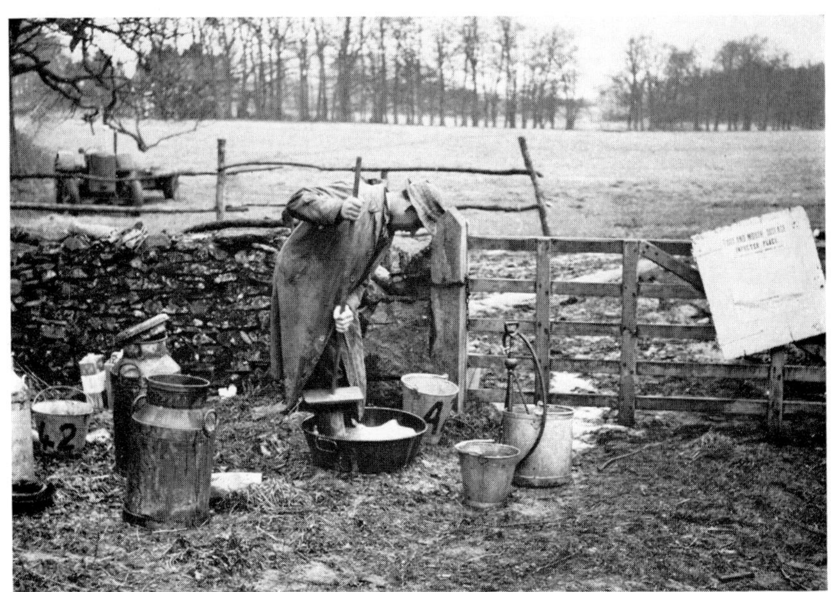

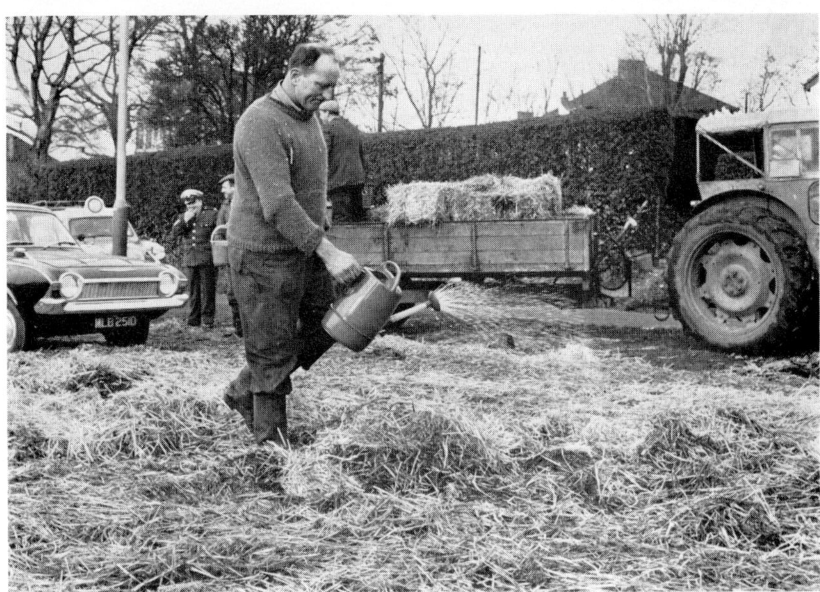

7. *Above:* Before entering the affected area, a farmhand takes the precaution of washing his boots in disinfectant. *The Field*

8. *Below:* Disinfectant being sprinkled onto straw strewn across the A.20 at Ruxley in Kent. One of many disinfectant barriers being put across the roads at strategic points in an effort to prevent the disease spreading. *The Field*

Britain markets were closed for a time, and again the people living in the stricken areas had a certain advantage. For the auctioneers and valuers there were kept busy at the alternative but unwelcome task of valuing animals for slaughter. So, too, with the veterinary surgeons. Some lost all their private clients but found full employment with the Ministry of Agriculture.

Hauliers forfeited about half their trade, though they still found employment in taking fatstock direct to abattoirs. Long-distance cattle-lorry drivers were forced to make extensive detours, carefully mapped out beforehand, to avoid infected areas. This particularly applied to traffic linking south and north, for while the A1 road was open for most of the period, it was closed for a time to livestock transport, diverted through east Lincolnshire.

Corn and feeding-stuff merchants found their trade in the affected areas dwindling to next to nothing, as indeed did every tradesman who supplied requisites to livestock farmers. Suppliers of farm machinery, however, had fluctuating business. Some farmers, as they received their compensation cheques, were attracted by the Ministry's inducements to switch to arable farming for a year and so started to equip themselves with tractors and cultivating machinery. On the other hand, service work on faulty machinery was virtually impossible on the farms. Some farmers brought their tractors and other machinery to the roadside for the mechanics to deal with, but others, sealed up on their farms, made do as best they could. The one branch of the agricultural machinery industry which found trade flourishing was the suppliers of heavy earth-moving equipment, in strong demand for digging burial pits.

As the epidemic developed, the towns as well as the countryside began to suffer. The country folk stayed away, their money ceased to circulate, and trade slowed down. Some towns, for example, Oswestry and Nantwich, became almost ghost towns. Nantwich, with over 200 outbreaks in a close circle around it, was like a place of the dead. Just before Christmas, too; and the effects were felt by such diverse interests as toy shops, grocers, television suppliers, hairdressers and caterers.

"There are no social functions on, so who wants a special Christmas hair-do," lamented one hairdresser. "And, anyway, the farmers' wives won't leave the farms."

"We can't get out into the country to deliver and install television sets, even if people came in to buy one," said a television dealer.

Country public-houses complained that they might as well close down. The recently-introduced breathalyser test had made customers very cautious in their drinking habits, thus cutting down the number of motoring visitors coming out from the towns, and local trade had practically vanished.

The banks noticed business falling off, and newspapers had to contend with a drop in advertisements. The *Chester Chronicle* estimated that by the end of November its fall in revenue from advertisements was more than £1,000 a week.

The police were naturally fully involved. They manned the control centres, stood guard over infected farms, provided escorts for heavy destroying machinery moving from one stricken farm to another, and generally ensured that the regulations were enforced. Men were drafted into the worst-affected areas from other districts, and the cancellation of week-end leave was a normal procedure. Their efforts were appreciated. At the control centre at Oswestry weekly bouquets of flowers were sent, anonymously, by "A farmer and his wife . . . for services rendered."

As soon as the magnitude of the visitation became apparent the Army was drafted in to help. Throughout November and December several hundreds of men from Western Command were engaged in the affected areas of the north-west, chiefly in disinfecting premises after slaughter. On leaving an infected farm, each soldier had to have a hot bath and a complete change of clothing and was not allowed to go on leave for a week. Army personnel were naturally delighted when restrictions were sufficiently relaxed to allow most of them home for Christmas.

Away from the heart of the epidemic army units manned check-points where disinfection mats had been laid across main roads, as far south as the Thames, until the Ministry of Agriculture pronounced such precautions ineffective. Others checked on the activities of ramblers and picnickers in the Pennines and Lakeland.

Figures published by the Customs and Excise on January 26th showed that the suspension of horse-racing cost the Exchequer more than £1 million in betting tax. The tax, on horse-racing and dog-racing, brought in £994,000 in December, 1967, as compared to £2,132,000 in November—a drop of £1,129,000. But the November figure itself had been reduced by the imposition of the ban on racing on November 28th.

Curious side-effects of the epidemic were reported. At Hawarden Airport, Flintshire, six out of ten flights to London were cancelled in one week in late November. Although fog was the official reason, clouds of smoke rolling in from the funeral pyres of cattle all around were an important contributing factor.

When Chester Zoo was closed, as a safety measure in mid-November, the animals soon began to pine for their visitors. Said a Zoo official:

"The trouble is the animals are used to having people watching and talking to them. A number of the animals are very much down in the dumps. . . . They will probably remain sad until the zoo opens up and people come to see them again."

Keepers did their best, by more frequent visiting and chatting, to supply the need, but there was great excitement among the animals when the zoo eventually re-opened.

[6]

Arguments

Controversy attended almost every aspect of the great cattle plague. As the toll mounted and the cost began to assume astronomical proportions, so the arguments about the effectiveness of the slaughter policy became more vehement. Farmers, press and Parliament all joined in.

As we said in a previous chapter the slaughter policy which eliminated rinderpest and pleuro-pneumonia has not been nearly as successful with foot-and-mouth disease. Indeed, apart from the quiet years, 1963 to 1965, the plague has shown signs of acquiring a firmer grip on our livestock industry since the war. Although slaughter remained, and remains, the official policy, it was as well to look at the alternatives. They are, of course, vaccination and cure.

In the *Western Gazette* (Yeovil) group of papers, to which I contribute a weekly column of country notes, I invited my readers in January, 1968, to tell of any foot-and-mouth disease cures they happened to know about. I appreciated, of course, that there was unlikely to be anyone left alive who remembered the farm cures in vogue before the slaughter policy came in, but I thought that some of them would be able to supply hearsay evidence from their fathers and grandfathers. And so it proved, though the witnesses were not as numerous as I expected.

A Nursteed (Devizes) reader wrote:

"Fifty years ago I was on a farm servicing a tractor when I noticed an old man whose hands and fingers were bent over like a claw. When I asked him why they were so deformed he said it was due to treating foot-and-mouth disease in cattle when he was a boy. It was his job to screw the hay into balls and push it down the cows' throats. That would have been well over a hundred years ago. They never killed the cattle in those days, and I have heard that they treated their feet with tar."

Another reader from Broadwey, near Weymouth, related that her grandfather came to the village mill in the 1830s, bought it in 1854 and remained there till his death in 1879. Attached to it was a small farm, consisting of several scattered fields, and here he kept a few cows, probably less than fourteen.

At some time, probably between 1862 and 1866, foot-and-mouth disease was diagnosed among the cows in one of the fields. They were treated by the local doctor, Dr John Williams Pridham, who was always keen to investigate any disease which presented a challenge.

"He kept the cows where they were and allowed no one near them, except one man and himself, and he was extremely particular about constant disinfecting. All the cows recovered, and no other animals, not even the pigs at the mill, caught the disease. I am sorry to say, though, that I do not know what the treatment was."

She added that in every field her grandfather had a shed of some sort as shelter for the animals. In the field where the outbreak occurred was a good stone shed, with thatch, in which the cows were treated. She rightly supposed that thatch could not have been the easiest material to disinfect.

Evidence also came from a Christchurch reader, who recounted what her mother (born 1870) had told her. Her grandfather had a mixed farm, with cattle, horses, sheep, pigs and poultry. One cow developed the disease. It was isolated, given a salt lick and treated with every care and attention. This cow recovered completely, and none of the other stock caught the infection.

My correspondent added, "Sick animals, of course, respond to care and kindliness. They seem to know that one is trying to help them. Comfort and a bucket of warm mash are great healers."

While I rightly realised that I could hope to get only this sort of second-hand evidence from my home readers, I welcomed a letter from a Fareham reader on his experiences in India.

"When we lived in Assam we kept quite a few livestock, including a herd of about 30 cows. The supervision of this herd fell within the province of the memsahib. My wife tells me that in fourteen years she can remember only one case of foot-and-mouth disease among our cattle, and that was cured.

The animal was segregated from the rest of the herd, and the sores were cleaned, probably with permanganate, which was usually handy. They were then treated with an ointment, the hooves being tarred and bandaged, to prevent licking. Treatment continued till the animal was cured. Although the herd was grazing on communal pastures with other cattle, no other animals caught the disease.

We do not remember the composition of the ointment but think it contained salt, tamarind, chillies, macerated neem leaves and possibly other local ingredients—but nothing exceptional, for all these things were readily to hand.

Sometimes we saw animals suffering from foot-and-mouth disease tethered in water, but I believe this was simply to prevent them licking their hooves. Foot-and-mouth disease must have been endemic then in India, as were also anthrax and rinderpest, but although I heard of epidemics of the two latter I never came across an epidemic of foot-and-mouth disease."

That is understandable, for a reason which I will discuss later in this chapter, but first let us look at a somewhat surprising story. To the general statement that after 1878 foot-and-mouth disease was not treated in Britain there is one important exception. This was on the Duke of Westminster's estate at Eaton Hall, Cheshire, in the 1923–4 epidemic.

The first outbreak on the Duke's estates occurred on Grange Farm on November 2nd, 1923, followed by another at Woodhouse Farm five days later and by one at Aldford Hall Farm towards the end of the month. At that time the farms were running about 400 cattle (including the celebrated Eaton Herd of Dairy Shorthorns), 300 sheep and 250 pigs, nearly all valuable pedigree stock. The second Duke of Westminster, who opposed the slaughter policy, pointed out to the Ministry of Agriculture that, as most of the surrounding farms had already had their stock slaughtered, his was virtually isolated. He therefore asked permission to try to cure his animals. In the end, the Ministry gave way. They insisted that it be clearly understood that the Duke would bear all expenses and any losses, without compensation, and that his flocks and herds would remain in strict isolation until the Ministry cleared them. This turned out to be at the end of the following June.

The manager of the Eaton Herd at that time was Mr H. Pakenham Hamilton, whom the present Duke of Westminster describes as "a man of infinite sagacity and experience". When, towards the end of November 1967, the great cattle plague was at its height, Mr Hamilton issued an eleven-page pamphlet, which had a considerable circulation, recalling his experiences of more than forty years earlier, as follows.

As soon as the Ministry's decision was known, the farms on the Duke's estate settled down to a state of siege, and the staff and their veterinary surgeons set to work on a problem with which none of them had had any experience. They were, however, not entirely without guidance. On the estate were a few old men who remembered how the disease had been treated in the days before the slaughter policy had been adopted. As a rather elaborate routine devised by the vets soon broke down, through the sheer numbers of animals requiring treatment at the same time, it was decided to give the older, simpler method a trial.

This consisted of syringing the feet and mouths of affected animals with a solution of salt and water, the solution being stronger for the feet than for the mouth. When the blisters on the feet broke, they were dressed with Stockholm tar. The tongue recovered quickly, without further treatment. In addition, animals which ran a high fever for a few days were given drenches to reduce their temperature. And milking cows which developed blisters on their teats had them dressed with ointment.

That was all. The rest was nursing and hygiene.

For instance, difficulties arose through some animals developing septic feet. Syringing them in their stalls created a wet mess underfoot, and dirt would enter the sores after the blisters broke. This problem was overcome by walking each animal to a hospital stall for treatment once or twice a day. Their residential stalls were kept well bedded with dry straw, and a rota of men and boys, operating right round the clock on a shift system, cleared away all the droppings and urine from the manure channel as fast as they fell.

"That was the answer," declared Mr Hamilton. "Keep the cow's feet clean for two to five days after the blisters burst and until the sores had more or less healed up, and all our troubles were over."

Blisters on the teats were troublesome, as they tended to seal off the teats and so had to be broken before the milk could be drawn off. However, the disease here provided its own answer, for as the fever developed so the milk dried up. The cows also went off their food for a few days, but as soon as the blisters on their tongues had broken and the sores had partially healed they started eating soft food, such as bran and soft meadow hay, and their appetite returned quickly.

As for the other cattle, the younger they were the less seriously they were affected, as a rule. Those aged between one and two years were bunched together in a clean yard where they had their feet sprayed, as effectively as possible, with salt water once a day (or twice, if there was time). For the rest of the day they were kept in a yard well bedded with clean straw. Only those which developed septic feet were caught and treated with Stockholm tar. Much the same procedure was adopted with young stock up to a year old, but the calves under two months received very little treatment at all. There just wasn't time to attend to them. Those which showed any symptoms had small blisters on their tongues but hardly any on their feet.

A bunch of rather wild Galloway steers, about three years old, received a somewhat perfunctory spraying with a salt solution. Here again, though, the disease assisted the treatment. Those which became ill enough to need proper treatment were in consequence quiet enough to be caught; those which did not, recovered on their own.

The big, heavy stock bulls promised to impose a problem. Fortunately, the only one of them which had septic feet happened to be a quiet old fellow who seemed to enjoy having his feet poulticed!

The pigs, a herd of pedigree Berkshires, did not go down with the disease until a month after the outbreak among the cattle. This was odd, for they were housed alongside and were fed with surplus milk from the cattle. Again, the treatment proved simpler than had been expected. Their feet became so sore that the pigs found it too painful to get up and run away. They simply lay there, squealing in anguish, when sprayed with salt water. When the blisters broke and the soreness passed, after a few days, they were eager to get up and look for food.

As for the sheep, it was never established whether they had foot-and-mouth disease or not. The shepherd certainly had an unprecedented crop of lame sheep, but none of them had blisters in the mouth. A procession of distinguished veterinary surgeons came to inspect them but could not make up their minds about it. Anyhow, all the sheep recovered.

Indeed, there were very few deaths among the Eaton livestock during the entire outbreak. Of the cows, two died. One was a very old matron who was on her last legs before she caught the disease; the other was accidentally choked while being drenched. None of the young stock died, except for two calves; and two calves in a herd that size is a normal mortality rate at any time. All the adult pigs recovered, though some of the sucking pigs died solely because their mothers had no milk to feed them.

The only long-term effects on the stock were on the milk yield. The cows did not return to normal yields till the next lactation. The ewes, which were pregnant at the time of the outbreak, produced a normal crop of lambs in the following spring. The sows resumed breeding normally.

The Galloway steers started to go off to the butcher about two months after they had had the disease and made excellent carcases. Several animals from the dairy herd, who had the disease in November and December, 1923, won prizes at the Royal Show in the following July. At a draft sale at Eaton on July 9th, 1924, 77 lots of cattle of all ages averaged £77 6s. 8d. each, which was an excellent record for those days. Top price was 550 guineas for the bull who had enjoyed being poulticed.

So the great foot-and-mouth outbreak at Eaton in 1923–4 ended with very little loss at all, though it gave the staff much labour and trouble for a few months. The essentials for treatment, Mr Hamilton emphasised, are good accommodation for the animals and ample labour to tend them in the first few weeks. Once the feet become badly septic, a complete cure could prove impossible.

To his little account of his campaign at Eaton, Mr Hamilton added a footnote on the prevention of the disease. Two old farmers in the village, who as boys had seen foot-and-mouth disease cured, pinned their faith on the prophylactic properties of gas tar. One of them was a neighbour who visited the infected farms on several occasions when the cows were being treated and who then went home to milk his own cows. The other was a farm employee who kept three cows of his own behind his cottage. He worked at the Eaton farms all day and milked his own cows morning and evening. Both men were generous in the use of gas tar as a disinfectant around their buildings, and both escaped the disease.

In the face of this evidence, the question arises: Would such a plan be practicable in Britain now?

It must be remembered that the conditions around Eaton Hall in 1923–4 were indeed exceptional. Most of the neighbouring herds had already been slaughtered, so that the danger of the disease spreading out from this centre was reduced. On a great estate such as this, it is easier to enforce complete isolation than on a small farm (though from the way in which local small farmers were allowed to visit the infected herds or were actually employed there it seems that restrictions were not very rigid). More important, perhaps, was the fact that the estate had a sufficiently large staff to give day-and-night attention to the victims.

Although we do not know what strain of virus was responsible for the 1923–4 outbreak, the strain which caused the 1967–8 epidemic was probably more virulent. Apparently wind-borne, it spread with a rapidity that surprised the authorities.

I do not think that curing foot-and-mouth disease, simple though the treatment may be, is a feasible alternative to the slaughter policy in Britain. It would almost certainly result, like the policy of vaccination which we shall be considering shortly, in the disease becoming endemic here.

In the matter of prevention, though, a closer examination of the properties of gas tar might be worth while; as also might an investigation into the merits of borax, which was widely used in Cheshire and the neighbouring counties in the later stages of the 1967–8 epidemic. Mr John Temple, Conservative M.P. for Chester, brought the borax treatment to the attention of the Minister of Agriculture in the House of Commons on December 4th. His herd of 200 Friesians were using it, he said, and it was estimated that at that time over 10,000 animals, belonging to well over 100 farmers, were also doing so. To that date, it was asserted, none of the herds so protected had caught foot-and-mouth disease, but it is impossible to say whether that record was maintained.

Borax tablets are homoeopathic in their action. Which means that, taken in small doses, they induce symptoms similar to those of foot-and-mouth disease. No doubt because of its resemblance to sympathetic magic homoeopathy is looked upon with suspicion by orthodox medicine. In this instance, however, there may be something to be said for it, although it is not suggested that borax gives complete and certain protection. Mr Stuart Ponsford-Raymond, of Raw Head Farm, Bickerton, Cheshire, who is chairman of the Malpas branch of the National Farmers' Union and who led the campaign in favour of the borax treatment, had bitter criticisms of the Ministry for not giving it a full trial.

Vaccination, the other alternative to the slaughter policy, became a focus for discussion towards the end of November, when the epidemic showed signs of getting out of hand. The Minister of Agriculture came under heavy fire in the Commons, and on November 28th, 1967, he announced that he had made arrangements for building up a stock-pile of vaccine, for use if things got any worse. As it happened, the vaccine was not used, which was just as well, for its employment would have been an admission of defeat.

The objections to vaccination are as follows:

1. The problem is similar to that of vaccinating against the common cold. Too many distinct types or strains of virus are involved, and no vaccine will give immunity against more than just a few of them.

2. The immunity given is only temporary. With cattle and sheep it lasts for four months in the first place; for about a year with subsequent injections. The implication is that cattle and sheep would have to be vaccinated twice in the first year, and thereafter annually.

3. This does not mean twice in the first year of the animal's life. The minimum age recommended for the vaccination of calves is six months. The calf is therefore unprotected for the first six months of its life.

4. Between the date of vaccination and the date when

immunity is established there is a time lag of from seven to ten days.

5. If the animal has already been infected, the vaccine is ineffective. As the incubation period of the virus is from two to fourteen days, there is no means of knowing whether it is present or not at the time of vaccination.

6. There is a minority of animals which carry the infection without exhibiting any symptoms. Against these the vaccine would be useless, and they would act as disease carriers.

7. The initial immunity given by vaccination to pigs is only four weeks. Indeed, protecting pigs by vaccine has so far proved an impracticable proposition. Yet pigs are often the type of livestock in which primary outbreaks occur.

In view of all these drawbacks, vaccination can hardly be claimed as an alternative to slaughter.

Nor would it be cheaper. Estimates of the cost of vaccinating all the cattle, sheep, pigs and goats in Britain to give them the best possible protection range from around £20 million to nearly £100 million annually. Until the 1967–8 epidemic occurred, the average cost of the slaughter policy was about £500,000 a year. So that even an annual recurrence of the huge bill for compensation for animals killed in the great plague —which Heaven forbid!—would be less expensive than annual vaccination.

Where vaccination may have a place is as a limited measure for throwing a cordon around an infected area. If this were done quickly enough, it could, in theory, prevent the spread of the disease, or at least give some measure of control. The speed at which the 1967 virus travelled, however, and the caprice with which it hopped about does not inspire confidence in the value of such a safety zone.

It is worth noting that in most countries where it is practised vaccination is regarded as a preparation for the slaughter policy. As soon as vaccination has reduced the incidence of the disease to a level sufficiently low for a slaughter policy to be adopted, the Government switches to slaughter.

Because of the gaps in the immunity given by any system of vaccination a policy of vaccination would be regarded by overseas farmers as evidence that foot-and-mouth disease was endemic with us. Immediately the barriers would go up against exports of our livestock. Against this argument it has been pointed out that the French, with the disease endemic though pretty well under control as a rule, manage to keep a good export trade going, even to countries with rigid regulations against the disease. It is true, but it is surely better to have the barriers left down than to have to concoct schemes for getting over them after they have been erected.

I refer now to H. G. Wells's *The War of the Worlds*. The Martians, it will be remembered, were vanquished not by any man-made methods but by disease germs against which they had no immunity. The situation has been paralleled in more than one primitive country whose inhabitants have fallen victim in large numbers to such diseases as the common cold and measles, which they were meeting for the first time.

The argument is valid in relation to foot-and-mouth disease, as numerous correspondents to the Press pointed out during the epidemic.

I quote Phyllis Gardiner in *The Times*:

"The policy of slaughter involving healthy and diseased animals alike can never allow of the development of resistant strains; thus the domestic cloven-hoofed animals, alone of all others, are denied by us the operation of one of the first principles of nature. . . .

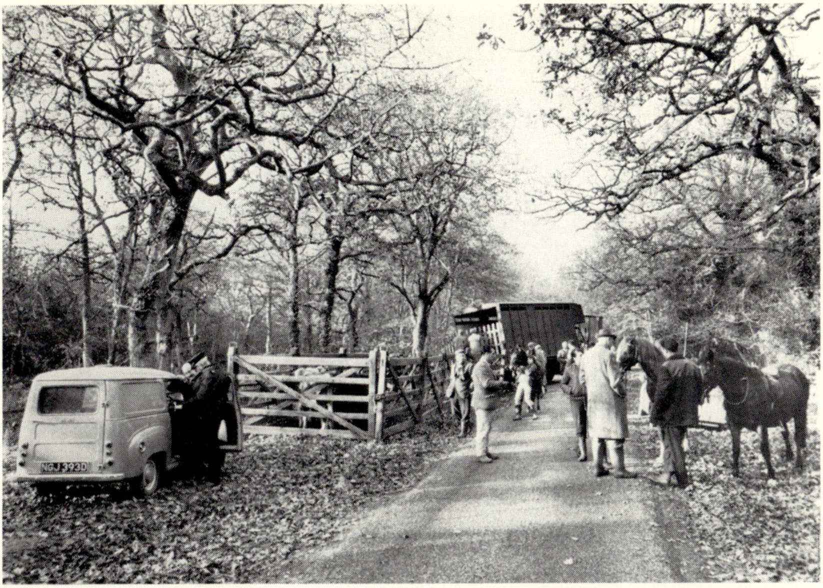

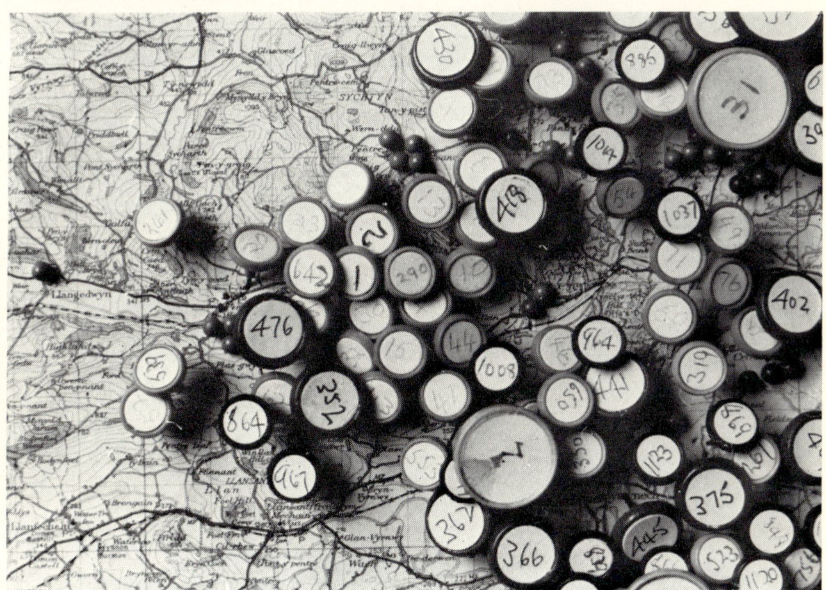

9. *Above:* The round-up of cattle and pigs in the New Forest, as a
   precaution against the spread of the disease. *The Field*

10. *Below:* Numbered pins at the Ministry of Agriculture Operations
    Rooms at Tolworth, Surrey, chart the course of the epidemic. Pin
    No. 1, near the centre, marks the first outbreak at Oswestry.

The Field

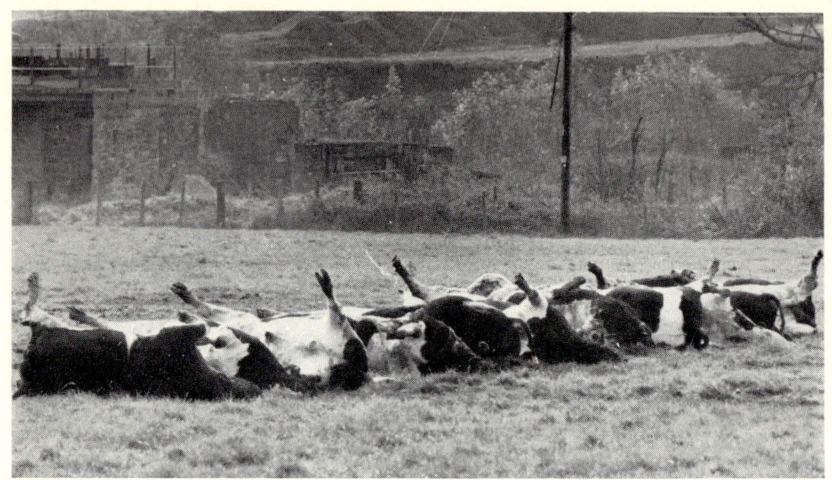

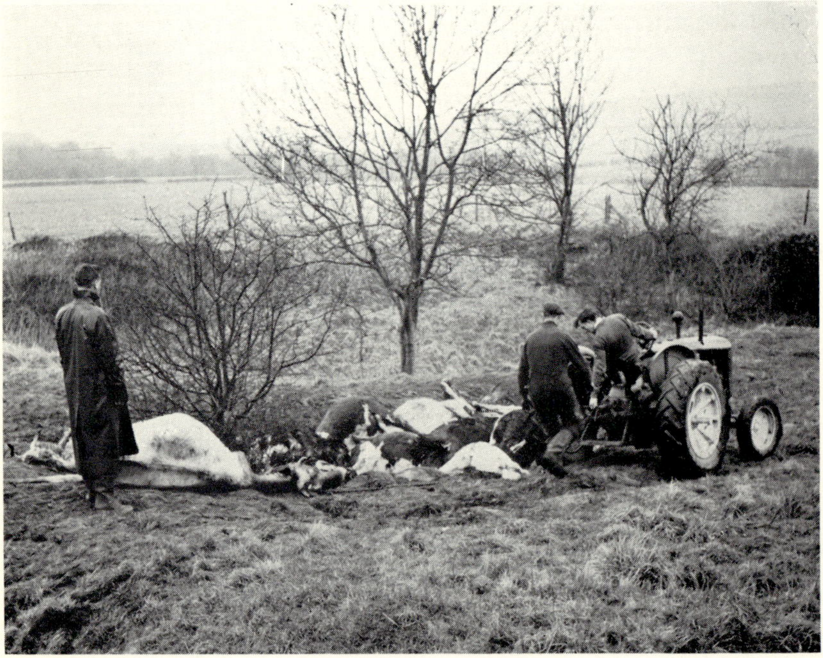

11. *Above:* Cattle awaiting burial after being slaughtered at an affected farm at Oswestry. *The Field*

12. *Below:* Slaughtered cattle being dragged by tractor to a disused quarry, where they will be buried in lime. *The Field*

The popular use of artificial insemination must surely make for animal populations of abnormally uniform genetic constitution, and the sires cannot be chosen for their resistance to disease. . . . It would seem that agricultural policy is running directly contrary to the operations of natural selection."

And J. Hopkins, in the *Farmers Weekly*:

". . . Is it not universally recognised in all afflictions, of both man and beast, the less they are exposed to any disease, thereby lowering their resistance, the more easily they succumb when thrown into contact with it?

While we have a national herd with this inbred and lowered resistance, with the disease still endemic almost anywhere in the world, it needs only one bird to fly in, or one bone to be imported into this country, and the door is wide open."

All that is completely true. So what? The logical answer to such objections is to expose our livestock to the disease, so that they can build up their own immunity. But how many generations would that take? And what would happen to our production and export trade in the meantime?

Which brings us to the contention that animals fed on organically produced foods, meaning those which have been grown without the aid of chemical sprays or fertilisers, are more resistant to the disease than the rest. Sir Albert Howard's experiments in India are often quoted as evidence to support this theory, but he was using improved stock in a country riddled with the disease.

In *Span*, an organ of the Soil Association, Mr Sam Mayall, of Harmer Hill, Shrewsbury, a leading exponent of organic farming, which he very successfully puts into practice on his large farm, wrote, in January, 1968:

". . . There is much misunderstanding as to the immunity from, or resistance to, disease that we may expect in a healthy stock that has been maintained in accordance with Soil Association principles. Though such animals have a very high resistance to the troubles normal to their environment, I have never believed that they are immune when brought into contact with a virus or bacillus which is entirely new to that environment. There are countless examples of this in human beings and animals the world over, and, to take one near home, the rabbits on my farm fared no better than anyone else's when myxomatosis first appeared.

Sir Albert Howard's experience with foot-and-mouth disease is often quoted, but foot-and-mouth disease is endemic in India, and it could be expected that his entirely healthy cattle would not be affected. Unfortunately the position is very different over here.

None of this lessens in any way my conviction that the way for a healthy life for humans and animals lies in the basic principles to which we all subscribe, but we must not let enthusiasm lead us on to expect too much. . . ."

Mr Mayall's herd went down with foot-and-mouth disease in the epidemic.

A minor controversy blew up over disinfection. Early inquiries to the Ministry of Agriculture as to what disinfectants were effective brought the reply that any of those listed under the Diseases of Animals (Disinfectants) Order would do. The list includes nearly 300 items, some of which were certainly less effective than others, but not washing soda.

A period of some confusion followed, during which it was difficult to get any reliable guidance from the various authorities. Then, in the last week of November, the Ministry's Animal Health Division at Tolworth, in Surrey, issued the following statement:

"We know that soda is more effective than other disinfectants against foot-and-mouth disease. We always use soda for general disinfecting on the infected place. But soda has disadvantages in some circumstances, for example when brought into contact with other materials such as clothing and leather and some metal, for example the undercarriages of cars. Consequently we have not recommended soda for general precautionary measures, for example at the farm gate.

Although it is true that other approved disinfectants take longer to kill the virus, we have always found them satisfactory in our long experience of foot-and-mouth disease."

The National Farmers' Union corroborated the advice that washing soda was as good as anything when used on materials which it did not damage, such as utensils, woodwork and rubber boots. It recommended hypochlorite solutions where it was liable to come into contact with human or animal skin, and carbolic disinfectants on roads and floors.

It added, wisely, "The general rule is that any disinfectant is better than none."

In the middle of January a Manchester chemical firm, W. C. Evans (Eccles) Ltd., brought out a new chemical, R–62 FAM, which they had developed specifically for fighting foot-and-mouth disease. Within fifteen seconds of contact, they claimed, this deadly disinfectant reduce 1,600,000 viruses to 25. Said Dr R. F. Sellars, deputy director of the Animal Virus Research Institute at Pirbright, to whom the chemical was submitted, "This is the fastest-acting disinfectant we have tested for reaction on the foot-and-mouth disease virus."

However, when the firm approached the Ministry of Agriculture it stubbed its toe against a brick wall. It was informed that all disinfectants on the approved list must, according to the Diseases of Animals (Disinfectants) Order of 1936, be derived from "lysol, coal tar or substituted phenolic types of chemical". There was therefore no point in submitting the chemical, which was not so constituted, for inclusion on the list, for the Order would have to be amended to get it in.

This was not to say that R–62 FAM could not be used as a precautionary measure. It was simply that, after an outbreak had occurred, disinfectants on the approved list *must* be used for the subsequent disinfecting.

That attitude seems fair enough, from the legal point of view, though somewhat hard on a firm that had concentrated on producing a foot-and-mouth killer rather than a general disinfectant. What strikes an observer as odd is that, at precisely the same time as it was taking this legalistic stand with Messrs W. C. Evans, the Ministry was widely advocating the use of and was itself using washing soda, which was *not* "derived from coal tar, lysol or substituted phenolic types of chemical" and was therefore not on the approved list.

Further argument developed over the use of disinfectant pads on roads and bridges. In the last week of November, when things were at their blackest, various local authorities all over the country took precautions to keep the disease at bay. The sensible thing to do seemed to be to lay heavily disinfected pads of straw or peat across main roads. In Devon the farmers themselves did this, manning each check-point with a rota of volunteers day and night. The Breconshire County Council, co-operating with The Dunlop Company, decided that disinfectant-soaked mats of a special plastic foam were more effective than straw or peat. Their lead was followed by Warwickshire County Council and other authorities, and the Dunlop factory was kept busy supplying the mats. On November 28th special instructions were issued to all army units in the Home Counties area to give priority to foot-and-mouth disease measures over all training exercises, and units were sent to man disinfectant points at bridges over the Thames.

The issue of the following notice by the Ministry of Agriculture on December 1st therefore came as a shock:

"The Minister fully understands the reasons that have led a number of farmers to get disinfectant pads or dips put on roads in certain areas. He is reluctant to dissuade anyone from taking any action which draws attention to the need for precautions. On the other hand, his veterinary advisers have no doubt that disinfectant at the farm gate is a far better precaution than indiscriminate use of disinfectant splashes on main roads far from the infected areas.

For this reason the Minister considers it should not be necessary to establish pads or splashes on such roads."

Naturally there was resentment at this announcement. The Berkshire branch of the National Farmers' Union described their reaction as "dismay and anger". Questions were asked inside and outside Parliament as to why the Ministry had needed four or five weeks to make up its mind on this point— weeks in which local authorities had in many instances spent several hundreds of pounds on road pads. No satisfactory answer was forthcoming.

The Ministry's announcement was a misguided one. Establishing road checks did nothing but good psychologically, even if its practical value was limited. Heaven knows there were too many people still ignoring the restrictions, even at the height of the epidemic.

For example, passionate couples in cars still parked in farm lanes after dark. Rubbish dumpers crept out into the countryside by night and emptied their trucks over the gates and hedges even of stricken farms. It took some time for everyone to realise that such callers as egg-collecting vans needed disinfecting just as much as milk lorries. Nor were farmers themselves immune from criticism. The wisdom of holding the Royal Smithfield Show in the first week of December was widely questioned. In the end it was allowed to go on, because of the immense contribution it makes to our export trade in agricultural machinery, but farmers were asked to stay away. Yet some of those who had already had foot-and-mouth disease on their farms attended.

The question of the general efficacy of disinfectants is still controversial, as new outbreaks continue to hit farms that have had the disease once and have been officially cleared. By mid-April, 1968, there have been thirteen such cases. It is true that they represent less than 1 per cent of the number of farms which have re-stocked, yet they are farms which have been given a thorough disinfecting and should be completely free from the virus.

The final criticism concerns the over-all control of the campaign in a visitation of this magnitude. Not a few farmers and politicians thought that a "Supremo" ought to have been appointed early on. Others advocated comprehensive leadership on a county basis.

In *The Field* of January 11th, 1968, Mr David Benson, who farms 210 acres at Aston Hall, Diddlebury, Craven Arms, Shropshire, gave an illuminating account of what happened when the disease struck his stock on December 1st. His comments are well reasoned and entirely relevant.

"The farm was stocked with 43 head of cattle and 202 head of sheep. The 210 acres is contained in a ring fence with an even rise of some 200 feet from the main Corvedale road to the northern boundary hedge. Most of the east and west boundaries are lanes giving good vehicular access.

Disposal

The diagnosis and valuation were quickly and efficiently done by experts in their respective fields. The chosen place for slaughter was at isolated buildings without electricity in the centre of the farm. This was conveniently near a suitable burning site, the possibility of burying having been excluded because of rock. The central position reduced to a minimum the risk of infection to neighbours. Or so I thought; I would not have made this suggestion had I had the full facts regarding the quantity of burning materials required, the vehicles and other equipment available and other requirements of lighting, access and timing. The result was chaos.

The veterinary officer postponed the slaughter to the following day, there being no light, and left no instructions when he went. Equipment arrived during the night and the following day, some burning materials never arrived, some broke down before arrival, and none reached the site because the access was unsuitable for the type of vehicle concerned. The slaughter was completed on December 2nd in spite of both guns breaking down.

The veterinary officer chose an alternative site for burning, but this, too, was inaccessible to the articulated vehicle and to other types of unsuitable vehicle used. He then decided to bury. This was completed by mid-day on December 4th. The site was chosen away from the boundary of the field and has left a monumental heap of rock.

COMMENT. A shocked occupier and a veterinary officer make a useless planning team. A practically minded expert with knowledge of the equipment available should be briefed by the owner and the veterinary officer and then produce a complete plan. The right man in this instance could have planned, laid down the procedure to be adopted and moved on to the next job in the two hours spent in valuation. This would have saved two days' muddled work when the risk of infecting others and the general unpleasantness were at their height.

Spare guns must be available. The choice of gun should be investigated. The normal human killer is more likely to stun than to kill. If it is Government policy to slaughter, they must have the proper equipment with which to implement it.

Disinfection

The infection area was small. The work was completed on the night of December 11th, six full days after the completion of burial. The 300 yards of farm road from the main entrance to the junction leading to the house and domestic buildings was deemed to be a "clean" road, although it had been continually used by the stockman, his tractor and his dogs coming straight from the infected animals. Stock for slaughter, clean vehicles, infected vehicles and men frequently used this 300-yard stretch and went off the premises without any form of disinfection.

A disinfecting point was established at the main entrance and another at the junction. The usual procedure was to park cars by the house and to carry out no disinfection when entering or leaving the main entrance. In general, Ministry cars used neither point and contractors' vehicles used the junction point only and then continued on infected ground to the main entrance. Men were disinfected, often in darkness under little or no supervision, at the junction point.

On Sunday, December 3rd, before the completion of burial, I was telephoned and asked to go down to the foot-and-mouth centre at Craven Arms. I refused and the veterinary officer concerned said that he would call by climbing the locked front gate. I thought the call was a hoax and rang back, to be told that the veterinary officer was on his way. He arrived as he had planned, having first told the policeman at the other entrance what he was doing. He left the same way with no form of disinfection.

COMMENT. Planned disinfection could have been completed in half the time with the same labour force. A plan could easily be made by the expert mentioned in my last comments and a further three days could be saved.

Disinfection, supervised by the policeman, should take place at the main entrance. Equipment should be provided, including a power pump. An adequate pump, worked from the tractor p.t.o., was available on this farm and forms part of the normal spray equipment used on many farms and by most agricultural contractors.

The contempt for disinfection shown by many Ministry men, including some veterinary officers, cannot be justified. There seemed to be a feeling that immunity from infection was obtained by seniority. If this criminal negligence was practised elsewhere it is small wonder that the disease spread so rapidly or, in view of the many miles that some of the workers commuted, so far.

Supervision

The labour force worked adequately under normal supervision but for most of the time the supervision was lax or non-existent. At least twice the appointed Ministry supervisor arrived several hours after the labour. A thoroughbred horse was sprayed with disinfectant for fun, an earth-moving implement broke the 3-foot-thick stone wall of a building, and the amount of work done per man per hour was less than half that done by the average farm worker.

COMMENT. If No Ministry men are available who are capable of supervising, the occupier of the farm should be told the plan and asked to arrange the supervision; or members of the disciplined services should be called in.

Excluding other officials, six different veterinary officers called on numerous separate occasions. On most of these visits, I answered identical questions, whereas the advice given by these veterinary officers varied considerably. No visiting official appeared to know what had been done or said by the other officials. I was never given any positive instructions or plan, and I am still confused as to the regulations.

COMMENT. It is accepted that the Ministry take control from the time of diagnosis to the time when disinfection is completed. This control would be simplified if a positive plan of action were made and recorded on a prepared proforma in an itemised sequence of work. On completion of any item the proforma could be signed and the time and date filled in so that any official and also the occupant could see the overall plan and what had been done by whom and where.

Such a proforma would prevent any repetitions and omissions of speech and work, prevent confusion and form a useful record of each case. A simple written copy of the regulations, if they exist, would be useful to all concerned. If they do not exist they should be published and an up-to-date stock maintained at each centre.

Finally, some general remarks. Throughout the twelve days of this case, every official was considerate and all endeavoured to help; some worked to the point of exhaustion. But there were too many of them, and the majority worked without co-ordination or direction in jobs to which they were ill-suited.

Too little has been done to stop the spread of the disease, and most of that which has been done has been done too late. A Ministry leaflet describing symptoms and how to guard my farm arrived after my beasts had been slaughtered. A leaflet telling me when I can plough, when I can re-stock, the exact position on taxation of compensation and other elucidation of *future* problems common to all infected premises would have been more apt.

Organisation

Action must be taken *now* to provide the closest possible scrutiny into an effective organisation to replace the present chaos.

It is unreasonable to ask a civil servant, and particularly a Ministry veterinary officer, to organise an area. What is wanted is a man who is known, efficient, capable and independent, who should always be standing by to take complete control of an outbreak of foot-and-mouth in every county. He should have agricultural knowledge and be a capable administrator.

He should be trained in the job and given complete control and over-riding powers in the event of an outbreak. He would be paid for doing the job, and he would only do it once. He would be a "supremo" and completely protected in any high-handed action he might think it proper to take. He must be savage, dictatorial and competent."

Though we may agree with Mr Benson that much needs to be altered before ever we are called upon to undertake another such campaign, it is worth noting his tribute to the personnel in the fight.

"Throughout the twelve days of this case, every official was considerate and all endeavoured to help; some worked to the point of exhaustion."

That opinion is echoed time and again by those who were in the thick of the fray.

We must also record that Mr Benson's views were indignantly challenged by several farmers in the farming press in the following few weeks.

For the greatest controversy of all we turn to the cause of the primary outbreak and the measures taken to prevent a recurrence.

From the very beginning, imported meat was under suspicion. In the last week of November the suspicions were sufficiently strong to prompt official protests from the presidents of the National Farmers' Union and the Farmers' Union of Wales. Both demanded the cessation of imports of meat from all countries in which foot-and-mouth disease was endemic. Within a few days, Argentina voluntarily suspended shipments to Britain, with the surprising explanation that the market price here for meat was too low. It was not until December 1st that the Minister of Agriculture announced the desired ban on meat imports.

The ban came into force on December 4th, and everyone naturally expected that it remain as long as the emergency lasted, although the initial period was for only three months. Early in January it was evident that the Minister was under pressure from various interests to relax the ban or certainly not to renew it after the three months were up, on March 4th. On January 10th the President of the National Farmers' Union sent an urgent letter to the Minister, requesting that the prohibition on imports should remain "until and unless a most searching inquiry can state categorically that they present no risk to our national herds and flocks".

As the Ministry had already decided on an official inquiry

into the epidemic and its causes, farmers felt sure that imports would not be resumed until the results of the inquiry were known. To their surprise and dismay on January 24th, Mr John Mackie, joint parliamentary secretary to the Ministry of Agriculture, refused to confirm this. Imports, it seemed, would be resumed. Most farmers felt, with Mr Gwilym Williams, the N.F.U. president, that this would be "an act of incredible folly and gross betrayal of the Government's duty to our farmers and their animals."

Throughout the rest of January and February the Ministry hesitated, subject to intense pressure from both sides. The farmers received powerful support from the press and from such organisations as the Women's Institutes, but arguments from meat traders and commercial interests in South America and other affected countries must have been equally formidable.

When the Ministry eventually announced its findings from the investigation into the cause of the primary outbreak at Llanyblodwell the critics became even more vociferous. It was established that Argentine beef and lamb were widely distributed in the district two or three weeks before the outbreak occurred. Boned lamb formed an important part of this trade, and the bones found their way to rubbish dumps, where they were doubtless gnawed by vermin. The vaccination scheme which is supposed to protect cattle in Argentina does not apply to sheep. Although, therefore, the outbreak could not be definitely traced to imported lamb from Argentina, the circumstantial evidence was very strong and, indeed, pointed in no other direction.

Rumours and allegations concerning the offending meat were widespread. Mr Grant-Ferris, the Conservative M.P. for Nantwich, declared in the House of Commons that he had been reliably informed that pressure had been brought to bear to prevent the proper analysis of the imported lamb. Later, the daily press carried allegations that the meat in question should have been condemned any way. On arrival in London from South America it was found, so the story went, to be infected with a food poisoning virus. It should have been destroyed but went to Wrexham by error. There an inspector who wished to test it was told by the Ministry of Health to release it for sale.

The Ministry of Agriculture stated that this tale referred to an earlier cargo which had been destroyed. Local people argued that it had never been established whether this was so or not.

The rumours were allowed to die a natural death, without the true facts ever being discovered or at any rate publicised. It does seem likely, however, that, during a protracted dock strike in Liverpool before the outbreak, an increasing shortage of meat in the north-western counties made the authorities a little less cautious than they might have been.

In spite of the storm of indignation which burst around Mr Peart's head when he announced his ban on Argentine lamb only, there was much logic in his decision. A ban on the importation of all meat from South America would make sense only if it were permanent. That, of course, was what farmers were hoping for, and still are, but unless the Government were willing to make such a decision there was not much to be said for imposing a temporary ban at all. Once the primary outbreak had occurred, the disease spread from this plague spot. It does not seem at all likely that other primary outbreaks were being started by other dollops of infected meat while the epidemic was in progress.

As a matter of arithmetic, Britain exports to Argentina annually goods to the value of about £23 million. Argentina supplies us with goods totalling £43 million. So the Argentinians come best out of the deal to the tune of around £20 million a year. Our exporters, however, are such powerful industries as iron, steel, electrical equipment, machinery manufactures, chemicals, insurance and shipping, besides which imported Argentinian meat offers better profits to meat traders than much home produce. So it was a battle of giants, which the Minister of Agriculture, like the shrewd politician he is, decided by a typical political compromise. He threw to the wolves the Argentine lamb trade amounting to only about £3 million a year.

Complained Mr Gwilym Williams, president of the N.F.U., "the decision can only be described as closing the attic window while leaving all the doors wide open".

[7]

Steps to Recovery

It is a measure of the resilience of British farmers that by the end of March, 1968, of the total of just over 2,300 farmers who had had their animals slaughtered, more than 1,300 had already re-stocked.

We have already mentioned Mr R. C. Hollinshead, of Minshull Vernon, near Crewe, who did not even wait for his farm to be officially cleared but started a new herd within weeks at a hired farm in Scotland.

Mr John Hoggarth, of Slyne, in north Lancashire, had 250 cattle and 70 sheep slaughtered on his three farms on November 9th, though an outbreak occurred on only one of them. He began re-stocking with cows and heifers in the week before Christmas, though with the precaution of domiciling the new stock on the two farms that had not actually been infected.

Mr Clive Rymond, of Benn Hills Farm, Sheepy Magna, Leicestershire, saw his herd of 67 milkers slaughtered on November 19th. The first of his new stock came in on January 3rd. Mr Rymond had invaluable allies. As chairman of the Warwickshire County Federation of Young Farmers' Clubs (he lives only just over the border from Warwickshire) he had colleagues who collected good animals for him, ready to shuttle them in at the earliest possible moment. Even so, he was a brave man to re-stock while the epidemic was still raging all around him.

96

As might have been expected, farmers who remained un-scathed by the epidemic were quick to offer help. On January 11th, after intense preparation of a suitable scheme, Mr Gwilym Williams, president of the National Farmers' Union, sent a personal letter to the 185,000 members of the Union inviting help in re-stocking. Each Union office compiled two registers of stock offered in its area. One was of animals offered for sale direct to farmers who had lost flocks and herds. The other consisted of animals from farmers who preferred them to be sold in special auction sales. The first register was sent to every N.F.U. county and local branch in the twenty-one affected counties.

Within a week, over 22,000 cattle and 17,000 sheep had been offered on the two registers. By February 20th, the totals had risen to 24,453 for dairy cattle, 18,805 for beef cattle, 36,306 sheep and 1,028 pigs. Transactions through the Private Treaty Register began on February 26th, and special sales were arranged later.

As already recorded, one of the earliest offers of help came from Her Majesty the Queen.

Registers similar to that of the National Farmers' Union were also prepared by a number of breed societies. Most of these were in due course integrated with the N.F.U. scheme, as were a number of charity funds, to which farmers and others gave stock or provided them at below market price. Among the earliest societies to act were the Ayrshire Cattle Society, which by February 12th had more than 6,500 cattle on offer, the Jersey Cattle Society, the Lincoln Red Cattle Society and the Sussex Cattle Society. The British Friesian Cattle Society, to which breed by far the greatest number of the slaughtered herds belonged, organised its re-stocking scheme through regional breeders' clubs. Other societies arranged re-stocking sales. The Pig Industry Development Authority also prepared registers of stock available, some at below market price, from its accredited breeders.

In Cheshire farmers formed the Cheshire Foot-and-Mouth Re-stocking Association to co-ordinate the activities of the various schemes and to re-stock on a group basis. The idea was to appoint a competent agent for each group, who would locate suitable cattle and make arrangements to have them inspected and purchased, rather than for each farmer to have to chase around making his own arrangements. Lord Woolley, former president of the National Farmers' Union, became the chairman of the working party which prepared the scheme, and the committee included representatives of the Cheshire branch of the N.F.U., the Cheshire Agricultural Society, the Country Landowners' Association, the Cheshire Association of Livestock Auctioneers, the Cheshire branch of the Farm Management Association, and the Cheshire Farmers' Club.

The Cheshire Farmers' Club was quick off the mark. Formed in early December for the one purpose, they quite early on linked up with a firm of London estate agents, who advertised for cattle in the farming papers and also approached many farmers direct. Within a short time over 20,000 head of stock had been offered to the Club. Having picked out the dairy cattle, the Club selection committee then visited the herds (in nearly every county in Britain), selected stock that they thought would suit their members and agreed on prices.

"I am pleased to say that the prices have been not more than £10 a head above pre-outbreak prices," said Mr Reg Roberts, chairman of the Club, when writing to me on February 18th. "We have one night per week for allocation. This is done in order of outbreak date, and the draw for the cattle is by ballot, resembling the F.A. Cup draw.

This has worked exceedingly well, and up to date all members with outbreaks previous to December 7th have received allocation, twenty have complete herds, and most have fairly large consignments. We think this is no mean achievement, as we have confined our purchases to young cattle up to calving-heifer stage, and we have not bought one beast that has not had an S19 injection (against that other cattle scourge, brucellosis).

Our figure for cattle allocated to date is over 2,000 and we feel that by the end of this month we shall more than double it."

The fact that the Club was able to secure the cattle at no more than £10 a head above pre-outbreak prices was good news and against popular expectation. The coincidence of the peak of the epidemic with the devaluation of the pound caused some confusion. Cattle prices climbed steeply in the autumn, and compensation rates, though trailing somewhat, rose in sympathy. Within a month, in November, they shot up by 40 per cent; that is to say, slaughtered cattle which would have been valued at the beginning of the month at £100 were valued at £140 at the end. Later the Government made some adjustments to the earlier compensation levels, to meet the situation.

To help in re-stocking, Overseas Agricultural Traders, Ltd., of Bury St Edmunds, launched, in January, a scheme for importing Canadian-Holstein in-calf heifers from Canada, as well as semen from first-class Canadian-Holstein bulls. Canadian-Holsteins are very similar to our Friesians, though considered by some to produce even more and better milk. The first batch arrived in England in May 1968. The price was estimated to be around £250 a head, which put this stock out of reach of farmers who wanted commercial animals at approximately the same price as those slaughtered.

The Government were rightly anxious that farmers should not be in too much of a hurry over re-stocking, particularly with dairy cattle. They feared that the very pressure of farmers seeking to replace over 200,000 cattle, most of them dairy cows, within a few months would inevitably force up prices. Across the sea, scores of thousands of young cattle which the Irish Government had successfully safeguarded from the epidemic were waiting to come over to replenish our herds, but they were mostly beef-type stores.

Before the epidemic excellent progress had been made in Britain with a campaign to eradicate brucellosis, or contagious abortion, in cattle. Many of the slaughtered herds had passed the test, and for these farms to have re-stocked with inferior cattle would have been a retrograde step.

From a national point of view, too, there was no cause for haste. In spite of the slaughter of so many of the most productive herds in the country, milk production rose steadily throughout the winter. In January, for instance, when the impact of the disease had been almost fully felt, milk production was up by 4·9 per cent on the figures for January 1967. It could be argued that the additional milk which would have been produced by all those slaughtered cows might have been an embarrassment to the Milk Marketing Board in its uphill fight to increase milk sales and maintain the price to producers.

Individual farmers, on the other hand, had to face the fact that the Government's compensation payments did not cover all losses. The Government's liability is to compensate for the full value of the animal slaughtered but not, if it is a dairy cow, for the milk it would have produced. Many farmers, but by no means all, were covered by private insurance policies against such consequential loss. Those who left it till the epidemic started before thinking about insurance found the increased premiums prohibitive.

To indicate just what it costs a farmer to wait for re-stocking, Mr Norman Coward, head of the Milk Marketing Board's Low Cost Production services, estimated:

"The average gross margin per cow in Low Cost Production herds is around £90 a year—or £7 10s. per month. This is the amount being lost every month by any farmer who is already geared up for milk production but who has no cows or less than he could manage."

So, again taking the example of a farmer who was milking 80 cows, he is dropping about £600 a month while his cow-stalls remain empty. But his overheads keep on.

The incentive to re-stock for those farmers who were protected by no insurance policies was thus very strong.

Farms saw their compensation money dwindling. There was the temptation, perhaps the necessity, of living off this payment and using it to pay off back debts. It was, of course, using capital for current expenses, but some farmers had little choice. And some farms, having got temporarily out of the red at the bank when their compensation cheque was paid in, thought long and hard about borrowing again to re-stock with interest rates at their level of 9 or 10 per cent.

With the idea of easing the return to dairying, the Minister of Agriculture on December 10th announced a £10 an acre ploughing grant for victims of the disease. That is, for every acre of pasture ploughed up for an arable crop the farmer would receive £10. So an alternative income to milk was offered for a year.

On March 11th, Mr Peart announced a further grant of £20 a head, to be paid on dairy cattle *not* replaced by October 1st, 1968. Again, the idea was to persuade farmers to grow a cash crop instead of producing grass for grazing by dairy cows. Thus a farmer who had had 80 dairy cows slaughtered and who yielded to the Ministry's persuasion to divert his cares to arable cropping, would draw a cheque for £1,600, simply for delaying re-stocking. He would also receive £10 an acre for all grassland ploughed, plus, of course, the normal price for crops produced.

It sounds a most attractive proposition, and some farmers found it so. Unfortunately the epidemic was concentrated on the prime dairying district of England and Wales. No place in the world is more densely populated by dairy cattle than Cheshire. The reason for this is that the Cheshire Plain produces some wonderful grassland, but it isn't at all suitable for arable farming. To plough some of the stiffer clays after Christmas (which was the programme dictated by the timing of the announcement) and then to sow with a late spring crop would have been an operation fraught with difficulty and trouble.

In no other region of Britain could an epidemic have hit so many pedigree herds, and the pedigree breeder had, and has, problems of his own. For him it is not a matter of buying in new stock from the most competitive market available. He has built up his herd over a long period of years, perhaps carrying on a tradition started by his father or grandfather. Some herds have introduced no female blood from outside for a lifetime, say, thirty or forty years, while their bulls have been carefully selected to introduce the characteristics which the farmer decided were the most important.

In such a herd the farmer knows far more about the ancestors of his cows than most of us do about our own. At the drop of a hat he can recite the pedigree and performance of any cow you care to pick out of his herd, quoting not only her lactation yields and the butterfat content of her milk but similar statistics for her great-great-grand-dam. To see such a carefully constructed edifice brutally destroyed in one smoking, stinking funeral pyre is a shattering experience. The British Friesian Cattle Society alone had about 250 members who thus went through the crucible. For them there can be no immediate and facile recovery. Sufficient numbers of cattle of the right breeding are not available. A few farmers may choose, and be able, to get back into the pedigree world by buying an entire herd, but most have to do it the slow way, as they did before, by the careful selection of individual animals over a long period of years. The period will be too long for the older farmers, though they will doubtless lay foundations for their sons and grandsons, for a human lifetime is too short for success in this pedigree business.

A somewhat similar problem faces the sheep farmer, whom perhaps we have been rather neglecting because of the sheer magnitude of the dairy disaster. Sheep become acclimatised to certain farms, particularly in mountain districts. It is a custom in most mountain areas for the purchaser or new tenant of a farm to take over the flock at valuation. These sheep, having lived on the place for generations, have acquired a certain immunity to its diseases and parasites. Farmers who have ignored this custom have found to their cost that new stock introduced from a distance almost invariably fail to thrive.

Now many farmers of the Welsh hills and the Pennines have been faced with that dilemma. Shall they run the risks of buying new stock from afar? Or shall they wait until there is sufficient local stock for them to build up new flocks gradually? Whichever way they choose, they have lost this year's lamb crop at least. No lamb cheque for them in July, August or September, 1968.

One of the more important repercussions of the great cattle plague was its effect on the breeding programme. Throughout much of the North and Midlands the artificial insemination service was widely disrupted for many weeks.

From eleven Milk Marketing Board centres a do-it-yourself A.I. service was operated. Disposable syringes of semen were collected by the farmers at the farm gate, in response to a telephone call. It was estimated that more than 30,000 inseminations were carried out in this manner, of which about 50 per cent were probably successful. Even so, a 50 per cent failure means a shortage of calves in the autumn of 1968.

To the layman the link between a foot-and-mouth disease epidemic and a shortage of meat may not be immediately obvious. It is easily explained when we remind ourselves that, to avoid the risk of infection, not a bit of meat from any of the slaughtered animals is ever used. That applies to animals which did not themselves have the disease but have simply been in contact with it or have lived on the same farm. All are either burned or buried.

During the great cattle plague the situation in some of the areas worst affected became so bad that abattoirs had to close down for lack of supplies. Those which remained open had to contend with a mass of constantly changing restrictions. For instance, an abattoir might be preparing to take, on the following day, a consignment of fat beasts for which all the movement licences had been duly issued. Then, just before midnight, a new outbreak on the farm next door would result in the automatic imposition of a standstill order for all stock within a radius of two miles. The farmer would be faced with the problem of feeding his fat cattle for a further indefinite period; the abattoir would be without work; and the customers for meat would be without supplies.

The FMC, one of the biggest meat-marketing organisations, which handles, for instance, about one-third of all the pigs marketed in the country, commented on the situation in the January issue of its *FMC News*.

"Diversions around infected areas—often major re-routing involving journeys of three or four times the usual distance— were arranged to get livestock to the factories and abattoirs. North-west Wales has been a particularly difficult locality from which stock had to be brought miles out of its way down the Welsh coast to reach the Midlands.

The whole trade in weaners became chaotic, and the repercussions will be felt for months.

Transport costs during the outbreak have risen considerably.

The Company has co-operated fully with the Ministry Veterinary Service in taking precautions against infection and observing the strictest hygienic standards. Field staff have refrained from visiting farms and have been working from homes and offices.

Despite the dislocation caused by this worst-ever epidemic of foot-and-mouth disease, supplies have generally got through, and so far there has been no real meat shortage. Some districts have experienced greater problems than others; the whole processes of marketing were widely disrupted, and meat prices rose sharply.

By-products operations received some setbacks. Approximately 60 tons of offal a week from Marsh *&* Baxter's Castle Bromwich factory had to be buried in a Birmingham tip instead of going to Stoke Bardolph (Notts) for processing."

Help was offered to affected farmers in a number of perhaps unexpected ways.

For example, N.F.U. Seeds Industries Ltd., extended its

favourable early-order terms for seed orders until April 30th. Normally the concessions offered end on January 15th. David Brown Tractors Ltd., offered a 10 per cent discount to all farmers who had lost their herds and wished to buy ploughs and switch from grassland to arable farming.

The Ministry of Agriculture promised that if farm improvement schemes were delayed as a result of foot-and-mouth disease an advance payment of up to 75 per cent of the grant would be made. The Royal Agricultural Benevolent Institution agreed to make up to £4,000 available from its own resources to help families experiencing severe hardship as a result of the epidemic and also to open a fund to receive contributions for the same purpose. The newly established Agricultural Training Board quickly planned emergency courses to train farmers and workers needing to switch to unfamiliar jobs after their herds were slaughtered. It made grants available to cover wages, travelling, meals and 75 per cent of the course fees.

The Treasury was as helpful as possible. For several months some anxiety prevailed about the liability of farmers to pay income tax on compensation for slaughtered animals. In the end, after close consultation between the Ministry of Agriculture, the Treasury, the Inland Revenue and the National Farmers' Union, agreement was reached and announced by Mr Harold Lever, Financial Secretary to the Treasury, in the House of Commons on March 5th.

The arrangements were a trifle complex, or at least require an understanding of income tax as it affects farmers, but briefly the provisions were as follows:

A farmer can, if he wishes, have his livestock assessed on a "herd basis". It applies to a herd of mature animals, such as of dairy cows, and its effect is to allow all these animals kept for production purposes (e.g. milk or progeny) to be assessed at unchanging value. That is to say, the valuation of production animals is not taken into account when calculating trading profits. Therefore, when animals are assessed on this basis, the compensation received for them when slaughtered in a foot-and-mouth disease epidemic is likewise not included in income tax calculations. For it is only an increase in value which is liable to income tax, and the value of these animals is, theoretically, static.

The Ministry of Agriculture considered that this provision took care of about two-thirds of the total compensation paid.

There remained one-third, paid in respect of young stock and fattening cattle and sheep. The value of these is naturally increasing all the time, and the increase is taxable income. Therefore compensation paid for them is subject to tax, to the extent that receipts for stock sold are part of the normal receipts from a rearing or fattening farm. Here, however, a concession was made in view of the fact that, if it had not been for compulsory slaughter, many of the animals would not have been sold in the current financial year. The Inland Revenue therefore allowed the receipts by way of compensation to be spread over the current year and three succeeding years.

All this seemed fair and reasonable, and few complaints were heard. The Country Landowners' Association, however, advised its members not to be precipitate about deciding to have their herds assessed on a "herd basis". There were cons as well as pros, they advised, and it might be as well to wait and learn something about the new taxation arrangements that the Government were known to be planning. And, in any event, farmers were to be given ample time for their choice.

The County Landowners' Association also approached, and was given a sympathetic hearing by, the Agricultural Mortgage Corporation with a request that, where a farmer had financial problems arising from an outbreak of foot-and-mouth disease, mortgage payments should be deferred. The banks, too, from which farmers in general nowadays borrow well over £500 million annually, were helpful, though they warned that borrowed money would be expensive.

In Rome on March 26th, Addeke H. Boerma, Director-General of the Food and Agricultural Organisation of the United Nations, congratulated the United Kingdom on its "tremendous efforts in fighting the recent foot-and-mouth epizootic". "Europe," he said, "is at present in a relatively satisfactory position."

Gradually life returned to normal.

On March 13th, Oswestry market, where the disease first struck, re-opened for cattle trade.

Paul Chambers of the *Daily Mail*, reporting the occasion, quoted, with a flash of inspiration, A. E. Housman's lines:

> "Graver notes the storm-cock sings
> to start the rusted wheel of things,
> and brutes in field and brutes in pen
> leap that the world goes round again."

On March 14th, the Duke of Northumberland presided over the first meeting of the Committee of Inquiry on Foot-and-Mouth Disease.

And on April 16th the first cargo of meat from South America was unloaded, to the protests of farmers all over Britain, at London Docks.

The world goes round again, and, without much doubt, in its circling it will bring yet another instalment of the Great Cattle Plague.

TABLE SHOWING OUTBREAKS OF FOOT-AND-MOUTH DISEASE 1922–66

YEAR	OUTBREAKS	CATTLE	SHEEP	PIGS	GOATS	TOTAL
1922	1,140	24,000	22,000	10,000		56,000
1923	1,929	69,000	26,000	33,000		128,000
1924	1,440	43,000	28,000	18,000		89,000
1925	260	9,000	8,000	3,000		20,000
1926	204	6,000	12,000	3,000		21,000
1927	143	5,000	3,000	2,000		10,000
1928	138	4,000	5,000	2,000		11,000
1929	38	1,000	1,000	1,000		3,000
1930	8	42	67	195		304
1931	97	4,000	6,000	1,000		11,000
1932	25	629	2,000	416		3,045
1933	87	3,000	3,000	1,000		7,000
1934	79	3,000	5,000	2,000		10,000
1935	56	3,000	7,000	3,000		12,000
1936	67	3,000	2,000	1,000		6,000
1937	187	9,000	15,000	7,000		31,000
1938	190	8,000	13,000	4,000		25,000
1939	99	3,000	5,000	4,000		12,000
1940	160	7,000	9,000	4,000		20,000
1941	264	13,000	11,000	3,000		27,000
1942	670	28,000	23,000	8,000		59,000
1943	27	1,000	2,000	1,000		4,000
1944	181	4,000	7,000	6,000		17,000
1945	129	3,000	2,000	6,000		11,000
1946	64	2,000	1,000	2,000		5,000
1947	104	5,000	2,000	3,000		10,000
1948	15	1,000	396	191		1,587
1949	15	733	373	2,000		3,106
1950	20	1,000	42	1,000		2,042
1951	116	6,000	4,000	3,000		13,000
1952	495	32,000	32,000	11,000		75,000
1953	40	1,000	5,000	1,000		7,000
1954	12	527	377	391	0	1,295
1955	9	664	713	24	5	1,623
1956	162	10,547	13,123	4,793	42	28,505
1957	184	11,284	12,885	6,221	20	30,410
1958	116	9,529	2,442	8,008	24	20,003
1959	45	2,251	2,284	3,179	3	7,717
1960	298	26,045	32,493	12,031	24	70,593
1961	103	7,078	9,813	8,149	9	25,049
1962	5	371	273	308	0	952
1963	nil	—	—	—	—	—
1964	nil	—	—	—	—	—
1965	1	154	—	—	—	154
1966	34	5,911	38,659	679	2	45,251

CUMULATIVE FIGURES SHOWING DAILY SLAUGHTERS WHEN THE FOOT-AND-MOUTH EPIDEMIC WAS AT ITS HEIGHT

DATE	OUTBREAKS	CATTLE	SHEEP	PIGS	GOATS	TOTAL
Nov. 10	207	20,033	12,141	13,545	5	45,724
11	252	22,444	14,557	14,343	6	51,350
12	277					
13	310	25,257	15,627	15,479	6	56,369
14	349	27,973	16,172	18,232	7	62,377
15	395	30,276	16,557	18,646	7	65,486
16	440	35,526	18,715	20,749	7	74,997
17	510	40,779	20,387	22,997	7	84,170
18	561	50,180	25,625	29,351	7	105,163
19	613	54,832	26,162	30,630	7	111,631
20	675	61,354	28,096	34,854	7	124,311
21	753	67,445	31,657	37,428	7	136,537
22	789	70,404	32,463	39,578	7	142,452
23	871	76,284	34,096	43,032	8	153,420
24	954	84,532	37,618	46,991	8	169,149
25	1,023	90,017	40,333	50,983	8	181,341
26	1,103	96,137	41,798	53,667	8	191,610
27	1,189	104,058	44,169	61,587	8	209,822
28	1,243	107,110	44,976	62,855	9	214,950
29	1,282	110,148	46,913	63,903	9	220,973
30	1,318	115,329	48,072	66,454	11	229,866
Dec. 1	1,364	118,885	49,293	69,884	12	238,074
2	1,405	121,069	51,344	71,406	14	243,833
3	1,460	125,315	53,527	74,071	14	252,927
4	1,504	128,974	54,572	75,058	14	258,618

5	1,557	132,699	55,265	76,558	14	264,536
6	1,604	136,086	55,518	77,184*	14	268,802
7	1,630	136,399	56,732	77,010*	14	270,155
8	1,657	138,391	57,219	77,692	15	273,317
9	1,697	142,058	58,837	79,511	15	280,421
10	1,725	144,232	59,438	81,113	15	284,798
11	1,759	146,918	60,861	82,264	15	290,158
12	1,789	149,011	61,960	82,778	15	293,764
13	1,817	151,183	62,738	83,504	15	297,440
14	1,849	153,891	64,274	84,391	15	302,571
15	1,878	156,412	64,838	85,772	15	307,037
16	1,910	158,730	66,540	87,637	15	312,922
17	1,934	160,564	66,962	88,487	15	316,028
18	1,951	161,588	67,194	88,814	15	317,611
19	1,974	163,143	67,429	89,545	15	320,132
20	1,998	164,730	67,981	90,759	15	323,485
21	2,016	166,073	68,998	91,707	15	326,793
22	2,035	167,766	69,217	91,972	15	328,970
23	2,055	169,722	69,792	93,691	15	333,220
24	2,075	170,974	72,524	95,178	15	338,741
25	2,091	172,598	73,422	95,535	15	341,570
26	2,108	173,583	73,734	96,218	15	343,550
27	2,128	174,737	74,450	96,615	15	345,817
28	2,145	175,772	74,758	97,353	15	347,898
29	2,152	176,413	75,009	97,773	15	349,169
30	2,165	177,192	75,271	97,778	15	350,256
31	2,176	177,895	76,263	98,119	15	352,292
Jan. 1	2,187	178,868	76,325	98,132	15	353,340
2	2,198	180,025	76,765	98,460	15	355,265
3	2,206	180,664	77,592	98,527	15	356,798

* Calculating error.